Illuminative Incident Analysis

Illuminative Incident Analysis is a unique method of team appraisal and personnel training. It has been formulated and developed by the two authors for use by care service staff. The technique centres around common crises. In a tutorial group, nurses, doctors, administrators and social workers select an incident personally experienced by one of them and are encouraged to clarify it through drawing. Drawing enables the group to reach more easily the deeper human and emotional aspects, the tensions, conflicts, and misperceptions that lie behind crises in teamwork. Why draw? One cannot illustrate 'Well I mean', or 'With respect' or other such cover-up phrases. Anyone *can* draw a lemon. Visual communication is basic to man, is more direct than speech and allows less opportunity for avoidance of important issues by emotional blocking. All those involved in the incident are represented first simply as pin-men illustrating the sequence of events. Then, putting themselves in the shoes of each member of the team in turn, the attitudes and roles of those involved are examined through exaggerating the initial drawings—often to the extent of caricature. When a staff nurse drew herself as a dustbin and a student nurse represented patients as so many cabbages passing along a conveyor belt, they revealed much about how they saw themselves and the people with and for whom they worked. More importantly, the drawings indicate how such incidents may be prevented and the team strengthened and developed

The drawings reproduced in this book were not made by an artist, but spontaneously by members of many tutorial groups. These real-life examples show that this is a practical and highly useful method of training people in critically important jobs.

The implications of this method for training in industry and business are immense, for what has been pioneered in hospitals can be done elsewhere to increase perception and self-awareness.

About the authors

Diana Cortazzi, educated at Summerhill, and graduating from University College, London, with a BA in Psychology, became involved in research on the problems of bombed families during the Second World War after a period of teaching, and then several years with the BBC, she began a career in the health service as a clinical psychologist. She established the only museum in the UK devoted to the early history of the mentally handicapped and is now mainly concerned with planning at St Lawrence's Hospital where she is Principal Psychologist.

Research into the co-ordination of services given to the mentally handi-capped led directly to the development of Illuminative Incident Analysis and a deep interest and involvement in management, administrative, and organizational problems of the health service. She is a founder member of ALP International, a group of management consultants, hospital and social service staff concerned to promote action-learning projects as first developed by Professor R. W. Revans. Her work includes a great deal of lecturing in the UK and overseas on action learning, mental handicap, and Illuminative Incident Analysis. Mrs Cortazzi is the co-author of *Action Learning* and a contributor to many books and journals.

Susan Roote read Psychology at Hull University, graduating in 1966. She then worked at Harperbury Hospital in Hertfordshire where she took part in two research projects on the use of teaching machines by the mentally retarded. Her work includes the teaching of her own and allied subjects to social service staff at local colleges and to health service staff in hospitals and clinics.

Since 1972, Mrs Roote has been working as Senior Psychologist at St Lawrence's Hospital and has, together with Diana Cortazzi, developed Illuminative Incident Analysis to its present highly effective level. She is presently concerned with the introduction of behaviour modification to train and manage patients at ward level, and with hospital management.

Illuminative Incident Analysis

Diana Cortazzi
Principal Psychologist
St Lawrence's Hospital, Caterham, Surrey

Susan Roote
Senior Psychologist
St Lawrence's Hospital, Caterham, Surrey

London · New York · St Louis · San Francisco · Düsseldorf · Johannesburg
Kuala Lumpur · Mexico · Montreal · New Delhi · Panama · Paris · São Paulo
Singapore · Sydney · Toronto

Published by

McGRAW-HILL Book Company (UK) Limited
MAIDENHEAD · BERKSHIRE · ENGLAND

Library of Congress Cataloging in Publication Data

Cortazzi, Diana.
      Illuminative incident analysis.

      (McGraw-Hill series in management)
        1.   Hospitals—Staff—In-service training.   2.   Health
care teams.   3.   Group relations training.   4.   Art
therapy.   I.   Roote, Susan, joint author.   II.   Title.
RA972.5.C67   658.31′24   74–23130
ISBN 0–07–084452–6

10   9   8   7   6   5   4   3   2   1

PRINTED AND BOUND IN GREAT BRITAIN

Contents

Part 2—Hidden depths

Part 3—Action learning

For Professor Reg Revans
thank-you is a small word
so we decided on action instead.

'Why,' said the Dodo,
'the best way to explain it
is to do it.'

Lewis Carroll: *Alice in Wonderland*

Foreword

This book is worth reading for three and a half good reasons. The first is moral: it dwells upon the earliest question ever recorded as being posed by human-kind. In verse 9 of the fourth chapter of *Genesis*, Cain asks 'Am I my brother's keeper?'–To which God might have replied 'Yes, you are. And what do you propose to do about it?' The fact that God is not reported as having answered the one question with the other does not absolve us today from the need to find our own answers to both questions. This book gives us particular insight about how to carry these social responsibilities, not only to our patients, but also to our colleagues: it is a book about teamwork.

The second reason is semantic. For Samuel Johnson described language as the dress of thought (Carlyle as the garment of thought), and we must not forget that many thoughts go around quite inadequately clad, almost risking prosecution for indecent exposure. But we can also turn Johnson's epigram inside out and suggest that thought is the garment of language, because (as those who are obliged to listen to much professional discourse are aware) many words can fly around virtually naked, clad in no thought whatever. This book therefore recognizes, accepts, and builds upon the sceptical paradox of Thomas Hobbes, that language is employed by men to conceal their thoughts. In its development of the cartoon, the illustration, the pictorial analogy, the visual image, the drawing, however crude and primitive, it strips away the veneer of literacy and tries to display human emotion as it was expressed in our infancy, and, if we may believe the historians of the Altamira caves, in the childhood of our race. If the great artist has nothing to say he leaves his canvas blank. The competent professor, however, will lecture for an hour to discharge his preliminary observations upon the nature of a vacuum. So, to understand the really important situations, where, as this book describes, the lives of the sick are at stake, it is most important that we rediscover methods of convey-ing to others what we sincerely feel and what we honestly fear, methods that are neither polluted nor corrupted by the ambiguous treachery of words. Nor is our need confined to communication with others: not a few of us might be happy to understand ourselves better, to know why we say the things we do, to interpret what we mean by them. And in the emotionally laden atmosphere of the hospital ward, it is for sure that we need a currency of exchange more rich and sensitive than the dictionary. The ward sister who, in one of Diana Cortazzi's self-disclosures, draws herself as a dustbin tells us just as much about her feelings as Wordsworth ever did about the dreadful effect of seeing his daffodils.

The third reason is pragmatic. This book is not derivative; it owes nothing to the doctrines of this or that particular school. It is the product of direct and first hand experiment, carried out by Diana Cortazzi and her co-author, Susan Roote, in the course of their professional work. Its sole claim to originality is that it induced her students (and others who helped to write it) to pay attention to their *own* experience, their *own* actions, their *own* feelings. In these days of pap-fed opinion, pap-fed interpretation, pap-fed commentary, forcibly piped through our cortical gullets by the illustrious and expert obscure of Fleet Street, it is reassuring to find somebody ready to return to a mode of thought not only admitting the individual but putting him back at the centre. What these exercises in self-help are reminding us is that even quite ordinary people —indeed, quite common ones—have feelings to express and interesting modes of expressing them. What other great books began as efforts by children to explain themselves to other children?

My last and third-and-a-half reason is educational, and is, on that account, not to be taken too seriously. But what one intelligent woman can do, others can at least try to do. What then might become of professional education—indeed, of education in all its forms—if we started to weave it from the ideas, illusions, hopes, images and other fantasies that play hide-and-seek in the misty labyrinths of the adolescent mind? Why should we be for ever governed by the dead and by the past? Why should not more of those called upon to teach our imaginative young throw in their lot with Diana Cortazzi and entice their charges, like the nuns of Bayeux, to embroider a new and instructive tapestry of our contemporary excitements? We are for too long cramped in our traditions of respect, teaching our students what our professors taught us. Is it not time we tried to learn from the students themselves? Diana Cortazzi and Susan Roote are making them both very eloquent and very persuasive.

Professor R. W. Revans

Preface

We are taught from our schooldays not to wash our dirty linen in public. We are suggesting in this book that 'dirty linen' should deliberately be used, not hidden away, for there is a richness of emotional energy in the shameful incidents that from time to time beset any group, whether family, organization or institution. . . . Not that the incident need be big enough to be described as shameful: trivial teatime gossip is equally productive of wasted energy.

The technique described in this book we have called Illuminative Incident Analysis to emphasize the positive aspect of throwing a bright beam of light upon the hidden aspects of teamwork that lie behind these occurrences. The technique relies upon three basic ideas.

The first concept is that the energy wasted in gossip, in anger, in blame, in the anxiety of inquiries and postmortems, can be harnessed to constructive action in team development. This is *The What of the book.*

The second concept is that drawing the incident, rather than discussing it, is both cathartic and constructive in understanding attitudes, role perception, and motivation. This is *The How of the book.*

The third idea concerns communication: the in-term of the 'seventies. Through the drawings and cartoons done by people who are analysing their own dirty linen, their own teatime gossip, we look at the realities which lie behind this deceptive, all-embracing term—at the pathology of the team. For it is our contention that a team can be sick and in need of diagnosis, treatment, and preventive measures, just as an individual member of that team may fall ill.

From the Illuminative Incidents, events which happen in the course of everyday life in an organization, we develop a Health Care Plan for the team. This is *The Why of the book.*

The illustrations are from the health and social services because this is our own field: the technique is equally applicable to other organizations and, indeed, to any circumstances where a group of people come together with a common objective.

Many of the incidents will seem familiar; almost all have been found in some form or other in a number of units, departments, hospitals, offices, and organizations in Europe and Asia, in Africa, Australia, and America. It is extremely unlikely, therefore, that any particular incident in this book can be identified as belonging exclusively to any one place.

▶ THIS IS A BOOK ABOUT OUR
MOST PRECIOUS RESOURCE: PEOPLE
▶ IT IS ABOUT PEOPLE WORKING
TOGETHER IN TEAMS

Diana Cortazzi
and
Susan Roote
St Lawrence's Hospital
Caterham
Surrey

Acknowledgements

We, too, have our Spider's Web team: we have been dependent upon many people for interest, encouragement, and energetic enthusiasm; and for support. These, we thank with particular gratitude:

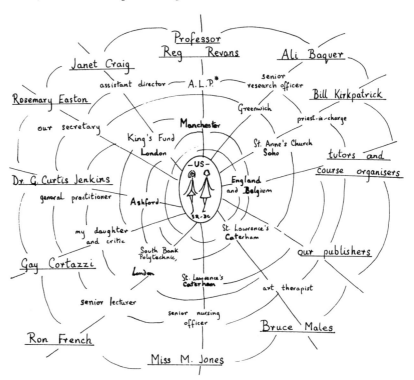

And thanks, too, to all our participants who so courageously brought their own incidents to be analysed: the drawings are theirs, the book really belongs to them.

* Action Learning Projects International.

THE WOBBLY JELLY

An old lady was sent home from hospital a day earlier than expected. She had no key, there was no food, no heating, no relative to meet her.

Nurse tells old lady and niece she is to be discharged home. Old lady very confused.

Social worker offers meals-on-wheels. Old lady refuses offer.

Ambulance man fetches old lady at wrong time.

Old lady arrives home coatless, keyless, foodless.

Jelly

Social worker - a Wobbly Jelly

Nurse in a Tizzy

ACTION NOW!

1. A simple, everyday incident where something has gone wrong and a patient suffered in some way.

2. Drawn by a training group to clarify the sequence of events and to lower the emotional temperature.

3. Turned into cartoon form to clarify the emotional needs of the professional team.

Illuminative incident analysis is a learning process which develops awareness

What is it?

DEVELOPING AWARENESS THROUGH THE TECHNIQUE of
Illuminative Incident Analysis means:
1. Taking an incident as a focusing point:
    ▶ an incident where someone has been let down, had a raw deal or suffered in some way;
    ▶ someone who should be served, or supported by a team or a group such as the family;
    ▶ the extreme example of an incident from a large organization with a team which serves is a patient dying in hospital; a small incident in a group—a grandchild smacked by an interfering grandmother.
2. Using powerful negative emotions:
    ▶ emotions arising from the fact that someone we should be responsible for has suffered or been let down.
    ▶ negative emotions, because we therefore feel guilt, anger, bitterness, fear or anxiety.
3. Re-directing these negative emotions to constructive actions:
    ▶ change of attitude
    ▶ understanding of roles
    ▶ sensitivity to others
    ▶ creative thinking
    ▶ new ways of working
    ▶ team development
4. Using drawings and cartoons rather than discussion:
    ▶ words are an alibi, words hide thoughts and feelings.
    ▶ drawings are like continental road signs—sharp, clear and compelling.
    ▶ drawing is therapeutic.

Part 1—The technique

1. The maps

Objectives to the chapter

1. To introduce the idea of developing awareness in a practical setting, through examples of
Illuminative Incidents and action that resulted
from analysis.
2. To discuss team development, the pathology
of the team and the concept of unused energy.

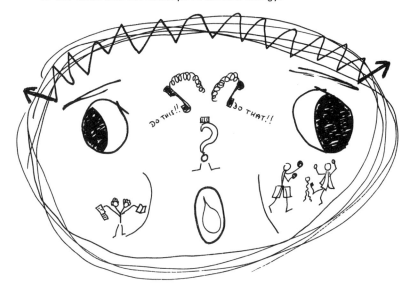

Where we get lost

How can it happen that neither patient nor nurse was told how serious an
operation was—and the man nearly died? What has gone wrong when a nurse
realizes that a colleague is wrongly instructing a student giving an injection—
and silently observes the mistake being made on a sick patient? What makes
someone in a caring profession serve cold mashed potato with hot custard
poured over it for pudding—to mentally handicapped people unable to speak
or protest?

Why does a teacher tell a child in hospital that his parents are coming to take him home, knowing they are not—and leave the nurse to deal with his outburst of temper when they fail to turn up? And why does the nurse then punish the child without discovering the cause of his bad behaviour? Who is to blame when a desperately sick man is sent to wait in a draughty hall at nine in the morning for transport—when the hall porter knows the ambulance is not due until the afternoon?

These are, of course, the wrong questions.

How can it happen? What has gone wrong? Who is to blame? Why? This is the language of negative searchings; it is uncreative. In the emotional climate of incidents like these, such questions can easily lead to blame, frustration and despair. At best, there is discussion on the need for more stringent regulations and procedures, more money, more buildings, more staff . . . tangible problems so often veiling the real roots of the incident. And at shop floor level, such discussions lead to further frustration, since resources remain always limited in relation to aims and plans; and regulations are sterile without goodwill. Technology in this decade we have in abundance: what is lacking are the skills of working together in a team in order to make optimum use of that technology.

It is important to realize that the people involved in these incidents are neither wicked nor malicious. The majority are highly qualified professionals, people who care, people of integrity and good-will who are desperately trying to do a good job. Often they work in difficult circumstances; sometimes, however, they are using the most up-to-date equipment in modern units.

It is when these individuals are unable to function effectively as a team that incidents happen. And used in a fresh way—analysed with drawings and cartoons rather than words—such incidents, far from being the negative stimulus to gossip or inquiries, to anxiety or blame, can become a source of strength in developing a team and in changing the attitudes and actions of its members. There is a wealth of energy in the emotions underlying a critical incident: anger, guilt, fear, bitterness—all potentially destructive and eroding, but capable of being turned into positive channels. Hence our use of the term: Illuminative Incident, which immediately switches attention to a positive possibility.

Our questions then become: how can we learn from difficulties and disaster, from trouble and distress, to locate the problems of team development in such a way as to strengthen the service given to both patients and colleagues? How can we use the situation which caused—and may again precipitate—a critical, an Illuminative Incident? How can we learn to use such incidents creatively, to make better use of our most precious resource—people?

The question becomes easier to answer when we look at the incident in terms of drawings, particularly when these are done by people actually involved in some way in the incident.

We have based this book on a technique of drawing such incidents and we take the reader on an exploration of this method to show some of the hidden depths of the iceberg that can wreck a team and allow these incidents to

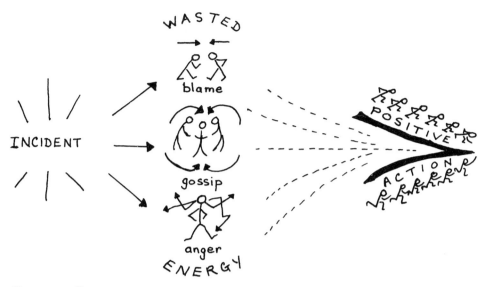

The energy diagram

happen. And, more important, to indicate how incidents may be prevented and the team strengthened or repaired. Drawing is only one method: we think it is simple and fruitful, and at the same time less threatening than other techniques such as role play or group therapy, which also have their place in team development.

The rest of this chapter considers in detail three different types of Illuminative Incident Analysis as an introduction to the technique.

The Pink Daisies

Incident: *Mentally handicapped women walked about in wet pants for some months—the targets of a 'who-does-what' dispute.*
A group of severely subnormal, incontinent women, in a hospital for the mentally handicapped, were being left wearing wet pants because the two groups of nursing staff looking after them refused to change them. 'It's not our job!' they both said.

The patients were in a special care unit where untrained nursing aides were assigned to teach them simple playgroup skills. Jaunty housewives, working weekdays only and not bothered about a career, the nursing aides were given pink uniform and therefore nicknamed 'The Pink Daisies' by the fully-trained nursing staff.

When these severely handicapped women wet their pants, the Pink Daisies promptly sent them back to the ward for the nurses to change them. But the nurses with alacrity returned the patients to the unit, still wet, with the message for the Pink Daisies: 'You're dressed up as nurses, in uniform— *you* change them!

For some months, the wet patients were shuttled back and forth in this way. In winter, they often had no pants at all. Neither side was willing to give way.

5

Although eventually this who-does-what dispute was solved, the resentment between the Pink Daisies and the qualified nurses remained for a number of years, the lack of teamwork affecting several different units.

It is one of our rules in Illuminative Incident Analysis that at least one member of a group exploring an incident should have been in some way, however remotely, personally involved. This is because it is our thesis that the powerful negative emotions that fester in the wake of an incident should be used constructively and that this is best done by those with an intimate knowledge of this, or similar incidents. In this case, one of the authors became involved by both sides as confidante, and having had some part to play in the early training of the handicapped women in this unit, was deeply concerned for their welfare. The drawings are, in this example, the author's.

What can we learn from this Illuminative Incident?

Roles
The first drawings were concerned with how each side saw itself and its opponent. It is interesting that the mentally handicapped women were spontaneously drawn as children, reflecting perhaps the protective attitude of the staff (including the author) who frequently refer to their patients as 'girls and boys' or 'lads and lassies'.

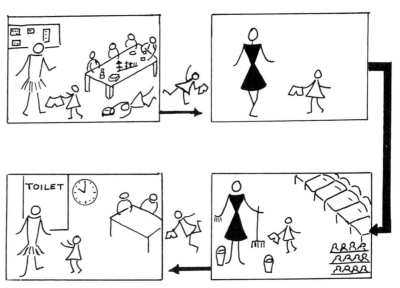

The Pink Daisies

The impact of the drawings made it obvious for the first time that each side is seeing itself as busy—if not overworked—with specific tasks on behalf of the handicapped women; and each side sees the other as relatively idle. The Pink Daisies are firmly convinced that the ward staff, having sent all their patients to various units, have little to do between meal times in comparison to their own hectic efforts to teach these restless women. The ward nurse, on the other hand, assumes that a special care unit must be concerned with basic teaching—and in her eyes, this means toilet training; why, therefore, send the patients back to her, when she has all the beds to make, the floor to clean, and a number of people who do not in fact attend any unit, to be washed, dressed and fed?

This is a basic problem of perception of roles which is frequently found in organizations where two different types of staff share a common client. The Pink Daisies therefore makes an immediate impact as an example of the type of incident we call 'illuminative'. And it is usually from such drawings of: How did each see the other? that the earliest insight comes to a group analysing an incident.

The team

Insight, however, is not enough: we are looking for active learning. With the Pink Daisies the next step came in the form of another diagram which explored the team concerned in the incident. This is how it appeared—the broken lines indicate poor communication.

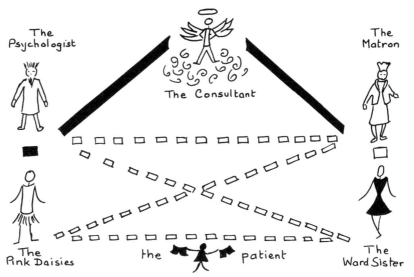

The Pink Daisies team

The consultant, it was realized, had *asked* the psychologist to start a special care unit and *told* him that the nursing aides (the Pink Daisies) working in the new unit would come directly under his care. The trouble began at the next stage when the consultant *informed* the matron (the principal nursing officer) that he had done so. She felt that a more reasonable procedure might have been consultation and discussion between the three parties concerned. Moreover, until this new unit was formed, the Pink Daisies had been on matron's staff. The one-way authoritarian approach to the matron then became a two-way affair of poor coordination and armed hostilities between her and the consultant. She next informed the ward staff that some of their patients would be attending the new unit—but in such a way that they in turn reflected her attitude to both consultant and psychologist, and to the Pink Daisies, who, now that they worked under the psychologist directly, ceased to regard themselves as nurses. The attitudes hardened when it became apparent that the Pink Daisies could have any equipment they wished, through the psychologist, while the ward nurses, ordering through a different channel, were heavily restricted and always short of play materials.

Although there was a perfectly reasonable explanation for this unorthodox administration of the new unit, the matter was never discussed with any of those concerned.

It is starkly clear in this new diagram of how the team was functioning that there *was* no team. Only a link between consultant–psychologist–Pink Daisies; and the latter, in the face of the attitudes of nurses and matron, grew tenuous. The Pink Daisies were forced into the position of having a boss who was himself isolated by events along one side of the hierarchy, but they were responsible at the same time for practical everyday dealings at the grass-roots level to the other side of the hierarchy, the nurses. And the patient–the mentally handicapped woman–is at the lowest level of the hierarchy–if not actually excluded from the picture.

So we have two approaches: the misperception of roles and the sick, malformed team.

Priorities

A new point for discussion throws further light on other depths behind the incident: what were the priorities of the various parties during the period of the Illuminative Incident? Individually, there would have been agreement that they had their patients' interest genuinely at heart. But at that time they appeared to the author to be as follows:

consultant $\begin{cases} \text{peace at any price} \\ \text{divide and rule} \end{cases}$

$\left.\begin{array}{l} \text{psychologist} \\ \text{matron} \end{array}\right\}$ territorial rights

$\begin{array}{l} \text{ward nurse} \\ \text{Pink Daisies} \end{array}$ $\begin{cases} \text{avoiding unpleasant job:} \\ \text{changing wet pants–} \\ \text{status} \end{cases}$

Who, one might be forgiven for asking, put the mentally handicapped women as their priority?

Knowledge, power and will

Another illuminating exploration is the question: who had the knowledge to change things, who had the power or authority to change them–and who had the will or desire to do so?

    knowledge: the student psychologist . . . who had *no power*

       power: consultant and senior psychologist . . . who had *no knowledge* and in fact denied the incidents

         will: *no one*

Knowledge, as so often in these incidents, is seen to be at the bottom of the hierarchy and the will, the impetus to change, has disappeared into a fog of apathy. To get any action from the team, all three are necessary: in this case, they were either non-existent or in the hands of the wrong members and so no action could be expected.

Action
From the analysis of this incident, many years later, evolved the idea of a 'spider's web' team, with the patient or client firmly at the centre. Each member of the team then directs his attention to the centre but at the same time supports, and is supported by the rest of the team, like the strong threads of a spider's web.

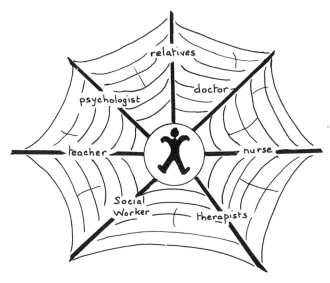

Spider's Web team

In its early days, working in such a circular team demands a conscious and constant effort; ultimately, communication between members becomes swift and adequate, and the feeling of mutual support is sustained in the lift of an eyebrow when passing on a corridor, or a brief word at lunch. It is a question of realizing that attitudes towards colleagues are as important as attitudes to clients and patients.

The Four Sons

Incident: *an old lady died and a ward sister was censured.*

The kindly, comfortable nurse was tense and bitter as she told her story.

> 'The old lady', she said, 'was over eighty, and had been bed-ridden in hospital for almost a year. But her four sons never seemed able to accept that she was both old and ill. Everything we did for her, they questioned; everything I said they wrote down in a notebook. Every visiting time they washed her and cleaned her teeth and combed her hair—even though we had just done it. . . . There were several things wrong with her and when finally it was decided she was strong enough for an operation, she died the day before this could be done. The sons reported me and there was an inquiry. They said I had neglected her.'

The inquiry asked: 'Why and How Did It Happen?' The kindly, comfortable nurse was exonerated. But six months later the bitterness still remained and so did the tension.

Words and pictures

To answer verbally the questions posed by the group of nurses from different parts of a large hospital and different levels in the hierarchy, is not necessarily to gain instant understanding and acceptance. Although, in fact, questions and drawings were simultaneous, the benefits of the latter are more sharply seen if the questions and answers are set out first.

▶ What did the four sons expect of the nurse? . . . That she would cure their mother and restore her to them

▶ How did they see the nurse? . . . As an angel of mercy

▶ How did the nurse see the sons? . . . As dominating her and interfering

▶ How did she feel about them? . . . Helpless

▶ How did the sons see their mother? . . . As a mother; comforting, reliable, someone to turn to

▶ How did the nurse see the doctors? . . . As not giving her information that she could pass on to the sons

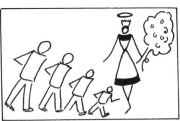

1. How the Sons saw the Nurse

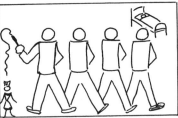

2. How the Nurse saw the Sons

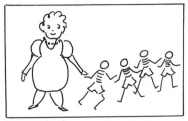

3. How the Sons saw their Mother

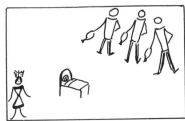

4. How the Nurse saw the Doctors

The Four Sons

To answer these questions in drawings or cartoons is to gain instant recognition of the problems, by the nurse herself, by the rest of the group, and by other people in different professions with similar problems.

Attitudes

The questions that interest the group analysing this incident are seen at a glance to be those concerning attitudes. The gaps in attitude are made plain by their decision to exaggerate the size of the characters in their cartoon.

The sons, drawn smaller than life in pictures 1 and 3, are seen to feel the need for a supportive, motherly person—whether it is their mother or the nurse. They raise the status of the nurse, depicting her as an all-powerful angel of wisdom, clutching the Tree of Knowledge; they see themselves—so the group felt—as small boys still, clutching their mother's hand. The nurse, however, draws herself as shrivelled and inadequate, both with the four sons and with her colleagues, the doctors. Already naturally worried about their mother, the sons' anxiety must be increased by their growing feeling that, since their mother is getting worse, the nurse must be inadequate: small wonder that their attitude becomes increasingly belligerent. Trouble was inevitable. To add to her feelings of inadequacy, the nurse sees the stark isolation of herself from the doctors who could support her. And so, the normally competent, kindly nurse, feeling herself to be small, helpless and unsupported, is scarcely able to give the relatives the support they in turn so badly need in their trouble.

Action
These drawings are extracted from a larger series constructed by the group in the four sessions they were able to spend exploring this incident. Changes in attitude and action taken following the analysis were striking.

First, there was the disappearance of all traces of bitterness: the nurse whose story this was had scarcely been able to pour out her tale at the first session, so great was her emotion. Now she was able to say with honesty—and in public:

'We dole out our information to relatives in a grudging and stilted manner, and place barriers between ourselves and the general public.'

The group said that through the analysis of the Four Sons they were made aware of the various interactions within the family; and of the way in which these and countless other relatives react to stress and sorrow. From now on, the nurse said, she would be sensitive to relatives' needs, and look upon them as needing support just as much as her patients did.

This was linked with the rapid completion of a book for relatives rewritten by one of the group involved in the exercise, with considerable insight into relatives' deeper and often unexpressed needs.

Another outcome was to start relatives' meetings: long contemplated but held up on various pretexts, they now actually took place.

One of the senior staff exploring this incident with the group now realized clearly the need for a nurse counsellor. Hitherto, he, like many others, had regarded the fact of seniority as automatically implying a capacity for self-support in times of stress. Now, the group realized that seniors might be just as much in need of support as their juniors. A counsellor was appointed.

Finally, two of the group started using this technique to solve ward problems as they arose, but in a modified form. They found it useful as long as they kept drawing. Unfortunately, they did not keep drawing—and found the group emotions difficult to handle in a purely verbal situation, and the meetings were dropped. It cannot be emphasized too strongly that it is the drawings that clarify, that are therapeutic, that relieve tension, that are remembered.

It is for this reason that we are trying to get away from words, particularly in tense and stressful situations.

It is not claimed that the use of this technique alone was responsible for all these activities. What does seem reasonable, is to suppose a sudden and effective release of constructive energy which had previously been misused on the negative feelings of bitterness and anger, anxiety, stress and guilt which had built up in this group of hospitals, around the whole question of relatives. The understanding achieved by the group in looking at themselves in the context of a highly emotional incident experienced by one of them, together with the released energy, evidently pushed concern into effective, constructive action. It was as if the frozen snow on a mountain slope had melted and turned into a powerful torrent of water, which was then harnessed to an electricity generator.

Both the nurse herself and her superiors commented on the therapeutic effect of analysing the incident in this way. It was not easy. It is difficult enough to be in a mixed group of colleagues, some from your own hospital, and to produce an incident which led to an inquiry as to your competence. To start with the sympathy of the whole group for the cavalier way in which you were treated by a group of relatives . . . and to end by admitting that these and other relatives deserve sympathy and support—this demands a rare degree of empathy and humility. The reward is in the relaxed approach of this nurse to her job and the richness she now gains from incorporating the relatives into her caring attitude.

The Wobbly Jelly

Incident: *an old lady was sent home from hospital to an empty house.*

The drawings in our first Illuminative Incident, the Pink Daisies, were straight-forward ordinary sketches. In the Four Sons, some exaggeration was deliberately incorporated by the group and the pictograms were deliberately used by them to show feelings of domination and of inferiority. Another enterprising group went a step further and chose to draw their characters in Walt Disney cartoon style. The full analysis is given to demonstrate the contrast both in style and in richness of subsequent action.

It was a young ward sister who told the story and gave it its original sad title: From Heaven to Hell in 24 Hours.

'Miss Smith', she explained, 'was a sweet old lady, always happy and uncomplaining. When she was due to leave hospital, I brought her into my office with her niece—her only relative—and though I was busy, I took some time to explain to them both that she would be sent home on Thursday by ambulance. They then both saw the social worker, who asked whether Miss Smith would like a home help or the meals-on-wheels service when she got home. She refused both services—she was an independent old lady.

It was only after the incident I discovered that she had subsequently told her niece she would be home on *Friday*, not Thursday—and the niece apparently took her word for it. Well, I was off sick on Thursday and it was operating day and we had a new staff nurse on duty. Everyone was

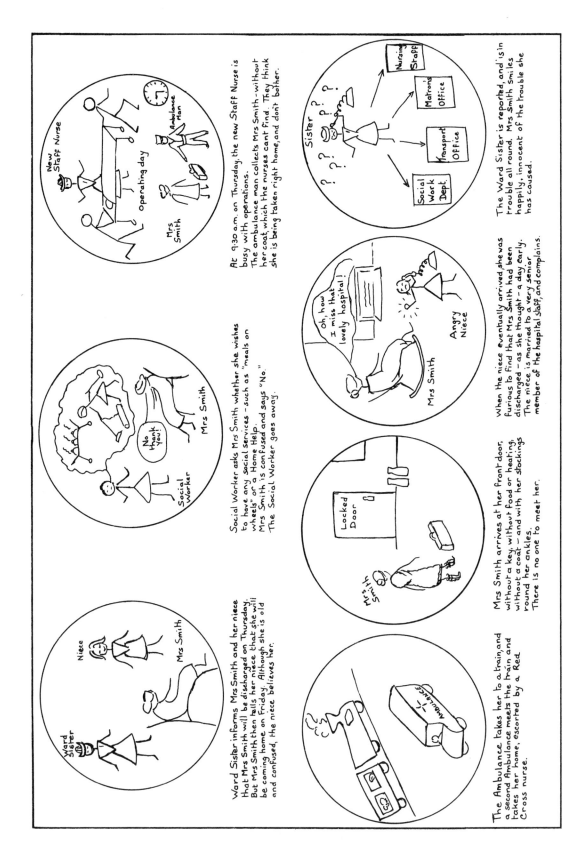

At 9.30 a.m. on Thursday, the new Staff Nurse is busy with operations. The ambulance man collects Mrs Smith – without her coat, which the nurses can't find. They think she is being taken right home, and don't bother.

The Ward Sister is reported, and is in trouble all round. Mrs Smith smiles happily, innocent of the trouble she has caused.

Social Worker asks Mrs Smith whether she wishes to have any social Services – such as "meals on wheels" or a Home Help. Mrs Smith is confused and says "No." The Social Worker goes away.

When the niece eventually arrived, she was furious to find that Mrs Smith had been discharged – as she thought – a day early. The niece is married to a very senior member of the hospital staff, and complains.

Ward Sister informs Mrs Smith and her niece that Mrs Smith will be discharged on Thursday. But Mrs Smith then tells her niece that she will be coming home on Friday. Although she is old and confused, the niece believes her.

Mrs Smith arrives at her front-door, without a key, without food or heating, without a coat – and with her stockings round her ankles. There is no one to meet her.

The Ambulance takes her to a train, and a second Ambulance meets the train and takes her home, escorted by a Red Cross nurse.

The Wobbly Jelly

13

terribly busy. Miss Smith wasn't due to go until the afternoon, but the ambulance men came at 9.30 and she went off quite happily with them, but without her coat or girdle. My young student nurse didn't bother much, as she assumed the ambulance would take her right home.

What no one on the ward had realized was that the ambulance only took Miss Smith to the station where she was met by a Red Cross volunteer and taken on the train journey (minus coat and girdle) and finally by Red Cross ambulance to her home.

It was Thursday and she was not expected. She had lost her own key, was shivering without her coat and her stockings were round her ankles. There was neither food nor heating in the house, because she had refused the social worker's offers of help.

Eventually her niece arrived, furious at the muddle, and reported me to the matron and to the senior consultant—although I had been off sick at the time. There was trouble all round. Far from being the happy angel of the day before, I was in hell!'

Drawing to cartoon
The first is a straightforward drawing, on the lines of the Pink Daises, telling the story in simplified form.

The second, cartoon drawing, came after a period of inertia when the group was beginning to blame the social worker as a superior youngster, fresh from college and 'knowing all the answers.' With a certain amount of prodding, the group agreed to consider how the young social worker might have felt. The following caricatures were evolved—and Miss Smith virtually vanished. She was no longer necessary.

Needs
These cartoons demonstrate clearly the practical advantages of delving behind the façade and abandoning conventional norms. From an attitude of: 'this is how it happened', the group turned to an important examination of the feelings of those concerned.

The young, inexperienced social worker is suddenly seen to be, not a superior person fresh from college, and knowing all the answers, as the group first thought; but a Wobbly Jelly, trembling and insecure and badly in need of support. In uncovering the façade, the group discovered for themselves the concept of the weak team member. And the discovery was made in such a way that she could now be seen constructively as in need of support, whereas hitherto she had been seen as 'useless'.

And the staff nurse, new to the ward on a busy operating day was illustrated by the group with considerable feeling now that the conventions were loosened. She is seen in a new light—not as an efficient person in charge of a ward and therefore competent at all times, but as a person 'in a tizzy', bewildered, giddy, unable to see straight, rushed off her feet. What they were probably not conscious of as they drew their cartoon, was the vivid indication of how the staff nurse could neither see, nor hear, nor speak: her communication channels were all effectively blocked by the chaos. She, too, had become temporarily the weak and ineffective member of the team.

14

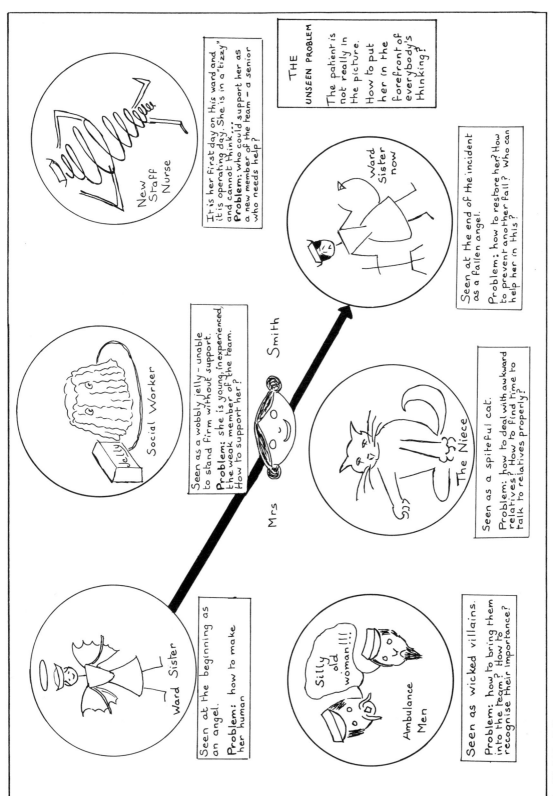

The Wobbly Jelly cartoon

This illuminated the fact that the weak member of a team could be a senior person. By illustrating the 'tizzy' in this way the group pinpointed a very common need of seniors and leaders: to have temporary support in times of harassing crises or peak rush-hours. It became evident that possession of status and a title did not necessarily bestow strength, competence and efficiency at all times.

The ambulance men, portrayed as Edwardian villains, were not seen by anyone as part of the team, although—since they knew both the time at which Miss Smith was due to be collected and the complex nature of the journey—their involvement might have prevented the incident.

And so, the precipitating incident, an old lady shivering in the cold outside her locked front door, has led this group to explore the subtleties and pathology of their team with insight and laughter; and to discover for themselves the deeper, more lasting and therefore serious causes of distress to their patient and to their colleagues.

Action
In this instance it took the form of a change in attitude, both in this group and in succeeding groups to whom the story has been told as an illustration.

Those who have laughed at these cartoons have told us that they can now spot a Wobbly Jelly in the most unexpected places: they are found in many different kinds of organization both in this country and abroad. So, too, with the Nurse in a Tizzy. And seeing the cartoons vividly in their minds, they have a different and more positive approach. The impact is immediate and compels action.

Why do we need a map?

Unused energy

Illuminative Incident Analysis as a technique focuses on team development; awareness of this skill is what we are trying to sharpen. The incidents discussed in this chapter indicate the importance of effective team work and of building on the strengths and weaknesses of its members. The powerful part of an iceberg lies hidden: we are using the visible tip (the Illuminative Incident) to guide us to the strength that is beneath the surface.

The team cannot, if it is to be effective, remain in a state of passive equilibrium. Its members must learn not only to work together and stay together, but to grow together and develop together. It must learn to support its less efficient members and its new members; it must learn to accept different ideas. It may be relatively easy to work together *today* when a project is new and exciting; but how can we help the team to stay together *tomorrow*—when the excitement wears off, when things get difficult, when there are anxieties and tensions, when work becomes routine and dull? And how can we entice the team to reach out constantly, to exert itself to achieve greater heights, to encourage its members to develop their hidden skills for the benefit of team and client?

What is important here is that the stresses and strains of a sick team are identified operationally, not just as another academic exercise. Each group is analysing an incident *in which one of its members has been involved*. Many quoted in this book may seem familiar since most occur in different places in a similar form in all types of organization, both in this country and abroad.

All the incidents demonstrate gaps: gaps in the service we give to a patient or client, or in the support we give to a colleague. It is through the exploration of such gaps *by the people familiar with or concerned in the incident* that constructive attitudes, alertness to the needs of clients and colleagues, team development and creative action can be effectively increased in a constantly changing system. It is a constructive use of negative energy: to develop a positive outlook in such a way that action will result.

The pathology of the team Just as one human being may become sick or diseased, or may have the misfortune to be born malformed—so may a group be malformed, or become diseased or sick. And just as the study of human pathology may indicate the causes of disease in an individual, so may a study of the pathology of the team suggest the form of disease that is attacking the team . . . a team, that is, that has been concerned in an Illuminative Incident of some kind.

It seems curious that we accept disease in an individual and seek practical methods of alleviation, of cure and of prevention, but seldom consider in a practical everyday setting the causes of malfunctioning in a team. Indeed, a protective complacency is likely to be found at all levels in an organization (except the most junior), denying the ineffectiveness of a team, particularly in some of the service industries or 'caring' professions such as mental handicap where there is no measure of success such as output in industry, or length-of-stay in a general hospital. So the team goes on, functioning below par, unaware of its own ineffectiveness. Even where success can be measured, a decline may be ascribed to material causes.

Yet a team *may* be born malformed, in that it does not include a particular individual or a representative from some group or profession concerned with the patient, or perhaps does not even include the patient or client himself. A team may become sick or diseased, in that some of its members may become ineffective, some may so dominate that others cannot use their own skills, some may become apathetic and opt out, some may 'not speak' to others, some may become so anxious or angry that they are not able to work with others, some may have to take a great deal of sick leave—and some may attempt suicide: it has been known.

We might quote St Paul on the body and its members:

> 'And whether one member suffer,
> all the members suffer with it . . .'

A sick person soon becomes aware of his illness, for he will have some physical indications: pain or fever, physical discomfort or sudden loss of weight. A team is less likely to be aware that something is wrong, for we have not yet discovered a parallel to the high temperature or the toothache that would send a team speeding to the medicine cupboard or the surgery. It is only when a drastic disaster occurs, and official inquiries roll over the ground, that it becomes obvious—too late—that all was not well.

In using this technique of Illuminative Incident Analysis, we are looking for something which is not easy to identify, let alone to accept. We are looking for diseases that may affect the welfare of a team; for causes of those diseases; and for preventive measures, for inoculations and immunizations that might protect the team from such loss of group effectiveness. We are looking, above all, for a *health care plan*, adaptable and flexible for use both in the here-and-now of the team and in its unpredictable future.

The team may not come out in spots to indicate to us the fact that it has measles; but we might learn to be alerted by incidents where the client suffers, to the fact that all is not well with the team, that it is sick in some way. Before the spots, the runny nose: our team may cry out to us with such phrases as: 'Who does he think he is!' 'What's it got to do with us?' 'I'd better not ask!' 'It's banging your head against a brick wall!' Little phrases behind which we might detect the early symptoms which will, with a certain inevitability, lead sooner or later to an incident of some kind.

This technique, of analysing an incident experienced by at least one member of a group, does succeed, when used in depth, in indicating symptoms, causes and amelioration. It allows the group to take a clear look at attitudes and perceptions, at individual responsibility and team-thinking. It allows them to appraise the support each member of the team receives from his colleagues. It does this in the practical, shop-floor setting, and in such a way that the development of more positive attitudes and constructive action is likely to result.

Dynamic development of the team

Never, ever, is a group allowed to apportion blame for an incident. Blame is a destructive mechanism, a negative use of emotion. The whole emphasis of this technique is on constructive examination of the gaps in the service to a client and on subsequent action, testing in another real, working situation what has been learned. It concentrates, therefore, not only on the client himself, but on the people whose job it is to be concerned with that client's needs.

It is not a question of sucking in one's breath in pious horror and saying: 'Ooh, how dreadful!'—but, in a positive way, of asking questions, such as the following, as a start to exploring the hidden depths of the iceberg:

'Where is the client?'
'Who is the team?'
'What needs to be done?'
'Who could help?'
'Who has information?'
'What information do I have that might help my colleagues?'
'How do we foresee tomorrow's needs?'

It is a question of locating the gaps in the service to *this* client who suffered today, in order to prevent gaps in the service to this and to all our clients of *tomorrow*. What critical information is needed, at which moment, by whom in order to effect changes in the service? How do we ensure that the changes are constructive and have a flexibility that will ensure development as other changes occur? What is X, the missing factor, that we could build in to our team to operate when rule books, memos and circulars fail? How does a team learn to work today while planning for tomorrow; to match *what might be* in the best of all possible worlds, with *what is*—with the reality of present resources, human and material?

Individual responsibility

The theme of this book is the team; and the team is only as efficient as each of its members. If one is sick, the team is sick. It is our contention that each individual member of the team must learn to bear responsibility for his colleagues as well as for his clients—in any aspect of his working life.
This may seem obvious in the case of senior staff bearing, one supposes, responsibility for the welfare and the training of juniors. But when one senior member of a team overhears another senior giving the junior a wrong instruction—and keeps quiet, perhaps it is less obvious. It is still less obvious when one senior who has a piece of vital information on a mentally handicapped man's ability to cross roads, thinks of another: 'Let her find out for herself!'—and he is run over; while another in a totally different situation is given the wrong injection. Nor is it obvious when the warden of a nurses' hostel realizing that one of the student nurses is getting quieter and quieter, asks no questions and takes no action—nor do the girl's friends. Until, one day, she is found unconscious from an overdose.

'Am I my brother's keeper?' may seem a question of purely ethical value: in a team situation the value is also highly practical.

We are not, it will be clear, discussing technicalities and expertise: we are concerned wholly with the emotional factors that can affect the efficiency of a team. It is easy enough to decide who should be in a team, who should be the leader or coordinator of that team, how often it should meet and what should be discussed. Easier still, one might imagine, to define the composition and duties of a treatment team. It is a matter of moments to draw up lists and issue memoranda about these things. What is remarkably difficult is to make that team into a living, creative reality that can not only deal with exciting projects or dire emergencies, but can also survive the monotony of routine week in and week out, year after year.

Well!

How *can* it happen?

2. How do we start?

Objectives to the chapter

1. To provide a framework in which to start an Illuminative Incident Analysis session.

2. To indicate some of the depths which might be explored.

3. To outline briefly some of the practical snags a tutor may meet, with suggestions which may help both tutor and group.

Preparation

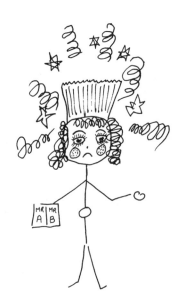

It may take a degree of courage for a tutor to introduce a session on Illuminative Incident Analysis with an incident in which he himself was personally involved. This is a challenging technique. It is not a parlour game.

Unless a group in whatever profession and at whatever level, can become personally involved in exploring its own world, in learning how to turn its own negative energy, as revealed by the incident, into positive action as a means of strengthening and developing both individual and team, the learning will be minimal. And the group is unlikely to become involved in this way unless the tutor himself deliberately takes a risk and illustrates his talk with one of his own blunders.

The technique is rewarding in direct proportion to the amount of one's own experience that is put into the analysis: personal involvement is vital. Moreover, the tutor who has previously analysed some incidents of his own, perhaps with colleagues, will be more vividly aware of those moments when the group may need encouragement or support. There is a time for dead-pan detachment and a time for gentle acceptance; a time for asking 'Why?'—and a time for declaring outrageously: 'I'll bet you felt like punching him on the nose!'

Such a statement did, in fact, startle the owner of one incident into an honest appreciation of a hierarchical situation, and relaxed the tensions and helplessness in the group: it led also to a new style of expressing the problems of the team.

This group, sketching a doctor standing pompously giving orders, suddenly saw him as a worm wriggling ineffectually and giving no support; and the visual impact of this cartoon compelled them to ask themselves the question: 'How to turn a worm into a tiger?' And from this, they spontaneously uncovered for themselves the concept of the weak member of the team: a concept which appears again and again at the stage of cartoon drawings.

This also illustrates a cardinal point: the keenest perception of the problem is there, in the team itself; and the richest solutions will come from the team. The tutor is merely there to enable a group to express what it knows and feels, perhaps subconsciously. He will, therefore, better fulfil his function as a leader if he has himself experienced a problem

The groups

While it is possible to analyse an Illuminative Incident with a whole class of students, it is more interesting to divide into groups of four or five and to allow time for reporting back to the class at the end of each session. With one tutor, a maximum of up to five groups is simultaneously possible—but frenetic. Groups of a single discipline are most common, but more insight into role perception, for instance, will be found with groups of mixed disciplines, since unfamiliarity with the background of the incident will lead to apparently simple but penetrating questions on aspects which might perhaps be taken for granted by a homogeneous group. For this reason, too, an outsider as tutor may elicit valuable aspects of the incident which would otherwise be missed. Groups of mixed levels in the same hierarchy have been tried with success; a learning process which may benefit both juniors and seniors. Groups have also been taken from the same discipline, but from different countries, and both medical and nursing administrators have demonstrated that this particular technique has a universal appeal.

Introducing the technique

This is largely an individual matter, and will in any case depend upon the purpose of the session and on the composition of the group. As a brief introduction, the authors usually describe Illuminative Incident Analysis as a method of learning from incidents, whether serious or trivial, amusing or sad, which happen in our own everyday work and which result in some kind of disservice to client or colleague. It is an attempt to make deliberate use of the negative emotions found in disaster or teatime gossip in a creative way; it is *learning by doing*.

We stress the analogy of medicine, which makes its greatest advances from studies of sickness and disease, from dissecting and analysing the pathology of the human body when something has gone wrong. And just as medicine studies the pathology and sickness of the body, so we are studying the sickness and pathology of the team—our own team—taking a moment when something has gone wrong as our first symptom.

Two or three brief examples are then given (but not analysed) as a trailer, selecting where possible one serious, one comic and one common incident. We might start with a story of information filed and forgotten, which is common to many professions and different organizations, and ask how it can happen that four or five experienced professional people could say: 'It's not *my* business!'

The story of Nigel, for instance:

> Nigel was a small boy in a long-stay hospital, who spent all day on the ward. A report sent by the psychologist to the doctor strongly recommended that Nigel be sent to school as a matter of some urgency. The doctor initialled the report and it was filed in Nigel's case notes by the nurse. One year later, it was found by the ward sister, who read it, and said: 'It's none of my business,' and put the file away. Nigel never did go to school.

We then go to a more serious incident and again ask how it can happen that senior people in caring professions see their job as caring, but not as communicating or coordinating information they hold. At every stage we make a point of firmly discouraging blame.

After these brief, unanalysed examples to signpost the group to the sort of incident that yields a rich harvest of discoveries, we then bring in an incident concerning ourselves. We may be brief, merely questioning the health, vigour and happiness of a professional caring team in which several members, including the speaker, could deliberately withhold information important to the welfare of the client; or we may use our own incident as a demonstration of one form of analysis. In either case, we make it clear that our actions or our attitudes have changed in some way as a result of analysing the incident.

Next, according to the type of session, we choose one recent example from a similar group and—having permission to use their story—illustrate one or two aspects of the technique of analysis. Whenever possible we show the original drawings, so that the groups are not daunted by imagined lack of drawing skills. *All the illustrations in this book are faithful copies of the originals.*

Finally, we comment on the constructive action taken as the result of a group analysing their own incident, for example, the Pink Daisies or the Four Sons— or some recent incident that fits the particular session.

We keep this introduction to the technique short, using illustrations rather than words, in order to start the more effective stage of 'learning by doing' as quickly as possible. With prepared handouts, large drawings or the use of an overhead projector, this introductory stage should not last more than twenty minutes. We then plunge straight into group work, armed with coloured pens and large sheets of paper.

The mechanics

1. Each group is asked to choose an incident *which has resulted in some kind of disservice* to the client or patient, student or colleague, and perhaps in problems for the staff which indirectly affect this service. The incident need not necessarily be disastrous or critical: an item of teatime gossip may prove just as good a starting point for exploring the pathology of the team. It is again pointed out that those with the courage to work on an incident of their own will learn more; but if a group is experiencing too much anxiety in the early stages, the tutor must be careful to leave a way out.

2. The first telling is often muddled and emotional; lacking in detail in some respects, it may contain characters who obscure the real issues and who are not necessary to the analysis. This may be the start of a therapeutic process for the owner of the episode; it may be a delaying tactic if exploration of the incident is not really desired. If a group is still at this stage at the end of ten minutes, the tutor may need to take the lead gently and encourage the group not to talk but to draw.

3. Next, some sort of drawing, pictogram, or diagram is constructed by one of the group—not necessarily the owner of the episode. The group should make suggestions, and by their questioning of what to draw next, again clarify the incident. The first drawing is usually on a time basis, or is a simple diagram of who spoke to whom. It is not important how this is done, as the object is only to illuminate the basic gaps as seen at the operational, overt stage of the incident. Nor is it at all important to be able to draw—few people can. A study of the illustrations throughout this book will make the point. Occasionally another member of the group, bursting to express his interpretation, may intervene or branch off into his own drawing. Comparison of the two versions can enrich the whole group's perception.

4. It is almost inevitable that some of the group will have been blaming someone or some deficiency in the material services such as money or old buildings or lack of staff—or quite simply, 'They'. It is important for the tutor to switch the emphasis. This may be done in a variety of ways—or the group may invent its own.

   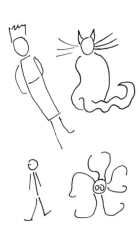

   It is always a help to suspend reality—to discard the first drawing and start afresh to illustrate the incident in the style of a Walt Disney cartoon, or a dream world. It is a greater revelation of the team's problems, for instance, to draw a nurse not as a pin woman but as a cat. Or, rather than drawing an awkward client as a pin man turn him into a manipulating octopus.

5. Groups vary in their approach from this stage on. Some are highly creative and need little help: others get into a rut, thinking round and round the same—apparently unanswerable—aspects of the problem. Here an outsider is useful, since in clarifying an apparently obvious point to a stranger, the group may see the incident in a new light, or express ideas of which they have been scarcely aware.

6. The group is encouraged to give the incident a title, and, again, this often highlights a basic problem, particularly for these groups who search for a

snappy or humorous title rather than for an accurate description of 'what really happened' e.g., 'the Wobbly Jelly'.

This may be as far as you will get in one session. If you have the opportunity for further sessions the *constructive* stages can be explored. But if you have to stop here, please consider point 9, 'Reporting Back'.

7. How does the group propose to strengthen the weak or inexperienced member of the team (who may turn out to be the most senior person) . . . or strengthen the Wobbly Jelly, or turn the Worm into a purring Tiger . . . or stop a train of administrators carrying cups of tea, telephones and type-writers from endlessly circling round on the circumference—and teach them to listen to their less well-off colleagues?

- ▶ Who could help?
- ▶ What could each individual contribute to the team?
- ▶ What knowledge has each member got locked away that could help his colleagues to help the client?
- ▶ Who could be in the team?
- ▶ Who might gain job satisfaction by being included in the team?
- ▶ Who needs to be thanked?
- ▶ In the best of all possible worlds, how should we communicate and with whom—and how much could we do here and now, if we *really* used our hidden resources?
- ▶ How can we stimulate people to *want* to communicate—since we cannot force messages to be read and understood and acted upon?
- ▶ What is X, the invisible factor that keeps a team positive and active, creative and continuously developing?
- ▶ What is a healthy team—and how do we become one?
- ▶ And, how do we stay healthy?

These questions can reveal a lot about the members of the group doing the analysis. For instance, a group of senior social workers were quite unable to imagine 'the best of all possible worlds' when discussing their incident, saying with determination 'because we are practical realists, we have no time for imagination'. Caught up in the daily rush, they had no conception of halting to take thought for the morrow, to plan for their clients' development or their own.

Although this is basically a discussing stage, the use of drawings and car-toons should still be encouraged, as they make the point more vividly and stay longer in the memory.

8. Finally, the distinction can be made between the *overt* causes which pre-cipitated the incident: lack of time, of staff, of equipment, of communica-tion . . . and the *covert* causes which the analysis has revealed: the attitudes, the human aspects of the team.

9. The stage of reporting back by each group in turn to the rest of their colleagues is very important, even if some earlier stages have been missed out. This is where the cross-fertilization, the sharing of anxieties and the release of tension when others laugh at your story and drawing efforts, are valuable consolidators of the learning which has already begun to take place.

Snags

A technique which is essentially a challenge to rethink one's role in a team, and which uses often painful incidents to alert a team to its own sickness, is certain to meet snags at some stage, largely arising from personal, or from personality problems within a group.

Group unwilling to split up

From the start, a group of ten or more may be reluctant or refuse to split into two smaller groups, despite the apparently reasonable explanation that a smaller group is likely to engage the active attention of each individual and therefore to experience the benefits of 'learning by doing'. If they persist in this, the tutor must respect the anxiety this shows, and try to give this group extra attention and support. It is not a common occurrence.

Vertical thinkers

A group may be quite unable to get away from the 'sand-in-the-works' phenomenon: a rigidity of thought and inability to escape from the original formulation of the story. There seem to be two levels of difficulty for the tutor.

'Who was responsible?'
Thinking in straight terms which demand a straight answer:

> 'Who was responsible? There should have been a memo (or an authorization, or a regulation, or a rule, or a procedure). He should have been there. She ought to have known.'

Often in a more senior group it takes some time to change this negative style of thinking, as it seems to be the accepted approach by some managers, but it is extremely important to do so. The 'ought to' and the 'should have' lead directly to destructive blaming, and the group—if left alone—will then disintegrate to the level of discordant gossip.

Part of the group's problem in analysis may be a natural anxiety. It is not easy to explore difficulties or disaster, however constructively, and if the incident is one's own, it does involve taking the risk of appearing to be inadequate in front of a group.

And so, at the surface level, the tutor can divert the group to another question such as who might have been in the team; how the various characters saw each other—and how they saw themselves; or to the priorities of each character at the time of the incident. Here, the value of the cartoon is seen, since it can easily lead to laughter and relax the anxiety.

'What do you want us to do?'
The tutor will inevitably meet individuals, and even occasionally a whole group, who demand to be told exactly what to do instead of discovering the delights of learning for themselves.

> '*Must* we give it a title?'
> 'Do we *have* to draw pin men?'
> 'Is this right? Is this how you want it?'

The problem of the vertical thinker (or more accurately in this setting, the vertical performer) has other facets, for it is not inevitably the older or more senior staff who react in this way when faced with a new technique. Evidence suggests that this attitude may already be present in a proportion of first-year university students. In an action-learning project in Dallas, USA, new students were presented with a similar situation in which they were invited actively to plan their own learning, rather than be passively taught. One-third were reported to have felt:

> . . . lost and confused with this unfamiliar structural
> design. Some responded with curiosity, exploring
> what could be done in the new situation. But others
> became passive, sullen or even violently angry,
> because they could not understand what was
> expected of them.*

In any large group there are likely to be a similar proportion of such 'vertical thinkers'. Normally they will be absorbed by their group, and occasionally, if this pattern is a form of defence against recent anxieties, may even change. It is more difficult when a whole group of vertical thinkers gets together; then the neophyte tutor might well be forgiven for experiencing a temporary loss of faith. Nothing, it seems, can persuade such a group to leave the motor-way and explore the unknown footpaths.

The authors so far admit defeat: others may be skilled enough to solve the mystery of the mature and often senior adult who, like a lost child, repeats, bewildered: 'Tell me where to go and what to do!'

Difficulty in suspending reality The cartoon stage, the Walt Disney type of illustration in which a rather woolly minded leader may be drawn as a sheep or as an amiable donkey, is vital not only to understanding the pathology of the team, but is an invaluable aid to memory and to action. It sometimes happens that a group—or a dominant member of a group—finds it difficult to suspend reality to this extent, but for others it is easy and enjoyable to do so.

> The group can only be offered the method: once again, the tutor *must not*
> impose upon the group, beyond encouragement to explore.

A group of medical administrators from overseas came up against a snag when using this technique. In their country, they said, it is forbidden to represent a person as any kind of animal at all—to do so, is regarded as an insult and is punishable, they could not, therefore, engage in Walt Disney drawing. Asked by the tutor to suggest their own alternative, these doctors produced some stimulating drawings, among them the invention of the 'Two-headed Nurse.' (See page 75.)

There will always be some who are unable to see the point of the exercise. To experience rebuff is the risk the tutor takes.

Sometimes, the group may have made some progress, but become suddenly blocked as, for example, in one session where they were trying to illustrate a

* Revans, R. W.: Psychosocial factors and nurse staffing. *International Journal of Nursing Studies*, **10**, pp. 149–160, 1973 Pergamon Press.

patient who was alive and one who had just died. The alive patient was happily drawn tucked up in bed; the group just could not think how to cope with the dead one, and ultimately the tutor remarked that someone had once drawn just a coffin or a headstone or a simple cross—and the group sprang to life again.

Had there been time, it would have been useful to explore this curious block, since most nurses find no problem in illustrating this particular point. If such encouragement is not enough the tutor may have to start drawing for them, while they make suggestions: this again, is rare.

'We've finished!'

A common cry, particularly from groups only marginally involved. Again, this may be a defence, if anxiety is coming to the surface. It may also be another aspect of a vertical-thinking group, a failure to grasp the richness of the technique, or failure on the tutor's part to explain clearly or to stimulate enthusiasm. It may even be another danger signal—as discussed in chapter 7. Whatever the reason, the tutor may be assured that it is beyond possibility that any group could finish exploring its own pathology, suggesting cures and devising ongoing preventive measures, in one brief session.

Again, use the hidden knowledge and energy in the group. The tutor may need to assume the role of naïve questioner, asking: 'Why?' or even: 'Why not?' . . . It may be a question of persuading the group to look at the way the patient was seeing the staff, was being seen by them, and was seeing himself: an exercise demanding both knowledge of human behaviour and a capacity for empathy. The hierarchical structure might be illustrated—in cartoons if the group will. The client's world might be explored in drawings and linked to the incident. The world of the owner of the incident might be looked at in the Utopian sense. Priorities, job satisfaction—there is a wealth of possibilities for exploration.

Individual responsibility

At a more complex level, it has to be realized that it may not be at all easy for some people to accept a philosophy as old as St Paul—but unfamiliar to many modern institutions: that the team as a whole is responsible for each member, *and* that each member is equally responsible for the well-being of the team. This is particularly difficult if that team exists within a hierarchical institution, and contains both senior and junior members. It is an all-pervading theme rather than a specific snag, but is extremely important.

It is evident that experienced, older, senior staff often find it hard to accept that their younger, junior colleagues may be as responsible for supporting them, as they themselves traditionally are for their juniors. Senior staff may not easily accept that support on both sides may include emotional support, concern for another individual beset by anxieties, personal or otherwise. The senior-junior responsibility is easier perhaps, in that it promotes a sense of power (seldom unwelcome); but the junior-senior responsibility almost certainly, if spelled out, evokes a feeling of dependency that may seem to some senior people almost a weakness to be concealed.

27

If some of this emerges in the course of analysing an incident, however mistily, the tutor can gently encourage the group to continue drawing—a greater safety valve than pure discussion. But the group *must not* be forced beyond its own pace.

The golden rules

To get the best out of Illuminative Incident Analysis, the tutor should remember nine important points:

Stick to your own story
... a story that has been experienced or at the least observed by, one of the group. Without personal emotional involvement, much of the richness will be lost.

Don't ramble on!
Extract the bones of the story.

Don't talk—draw!
Even feelings, most of all feelings. Stick at it: the more difficult to express in drawing the more rewarding the effort will be.

Draw from the stomach!
Suspend intelligence and reason—you will learn an astonishing amount!

Try twice ...
The second (or even the third) drawing is the one which reveals most.

Remember the safety valves
Drawings and laughter are essential safety valves for emotions. Words are a smoke screen.

Take a risk!
Be daring. Don't be afraid to make a fool of yourself.

Do not *apportion blame*
Stop all attempts to 'find the guilty person, the one responsible' immediately. This is negative. It will inhibit the development of the incident into pictorial form and constructive conclusions.

Signpost ahead!
Always end on a constructive note. The whole point of Illuminative Incident Analysis is to lead to a fresh look at oneself and one's colleagues in the team. See that you use the 'Energy Diagram' in chapter 1 positively.

Teaching notes

We learnt the hard way. You will make your own mistakes, but at least this may help you avoid ours.

► In choosing a story: make sure the owner of the incident is familiar enough with it, otherwise the group will become frustrated by their ignorance.
► Large sheets of paper will give the best results and so will the offer of a

selection of coloured felt pens. We always use sheets of paper 20 x 15 in, since the feeling of space encourages free expression of feelings in the drawings.

▶ Make it informal: some of our best sessions were done sprawled on the floor.

▶ Avoid the trap of leaving your own examples lying around—some groups may be tempted to imitate the style rather than use their own imagination. One session of ours even started by drawing eight circles with eight boxes underneath exactly as in 'Wobbly Jelly', and tried to fit their own story into this pattern!

▶ Inevitably, some will get bogged down. Keep an eye on things so that you can step in as soon as they do get stuck, armed with fresh paper and suggestions for a new look. It may help to change the group's artist. Or get some people from a different group to listen and help.

▶ On the other hand be prepared to be told: 'Go away—we're quite happy!'

▶ It won't go down equally well with everybody—don't expect it to. It's not always your failure.

▶ Reporting back is a good way of ending on an optimistic note and is an important part of group learning.

▶ This seems to be a good way to tackle Illuminative Incident Analysis—but *you* may find a better one. Develop your own style.

Remember!

Learn by doing—

don't try to teach

3. Why draw?

Objectives to the chapter

1. To present various illustrations of the impact of drawing as a shorthand form to clarify the feelings and emotions that lie behind incidents.

2. To suggest a socially acceptable form of revealing unacceptable attitudes.

3. To indicate ways of ameliorating the sickness in a team.

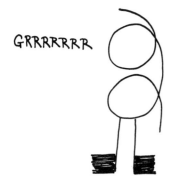

GRRRRRR

It is just because there is a great deal of emotion and tension hovering in the air that verbal discussion of an Illuminative Incident is likely to be abortive. A smoke screen will be created around feelings too intense or painful, and the objectives of the exercise will be lost. There will be blocks, alibis, defences and, almost certainly, indignation and blame. To reach the deeper human aspects, the behaviour and attitudes, the misperceptions that lie behind the incident, will be difficult. There are other good reasons for drawing which we discuss and illustrate in this chapter.

Clarification

. . . of the incident

Lines, unlike words, will not hide woolly thinking. It is just not possible to draw the: 'Well, I mean . . .', the: 'Sort of . . .', the: 'You see . . .', or the discursive meandering phrases that make our journeys into each others' minds as tiring as travelling in a train during a 'go-slow' edict. Indeed, the inability to reconstruct an incident in the form of a pin-man drawing, however simple, may in itself suggest a facet of communication worth exploring. It is astonishing how many key personnel in a coordinating position have difficulty in outlining an event in concise and simple terms—even in professions where such communication may frequently be a matter of great urgency. Analysis by drawing may be an educative process in this respect.

. . . of feelings

Reality is easily hidden behind words, but difficult to disguise in pencil lines. Certainly, feelings will be more accurately indicated in a drawing, as every art therapist knows; and ultimately, it is feelings that interest us. There, the energy lies. The decision as to where to place characters on the paper may clarify their importance in the incident. It also clarifies which people were close to, or removed from, the client. Indeed, there are times when the client does not appear in the drawing at all, in itself a clarification.

. . . of problems

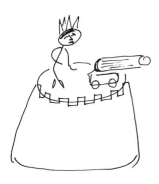

A unit, an office, a person may be isolated: it frequently happens that those concerned are genuinely unaware of this until the moment of constructing the drawing. The team may see that their key person is not coordinating or communicating effectively: the thought may have been there, unspoken; but the drawing, consciously or subconsciously, will often focus on this dramatically. The consultant in his fortress, for instance, is not only alone, but is isolating himself effectively with his cannon—frightened of whom? His colleagues? His team? His patient? Only by learning to put ourselves in his shoes can we begin to feel the answer.

Alleviation

It is not only as expressions of a basic problem that these apparently silly drawings have value. The cartoon becomes a form of shorthand: a simple formula which sticks in the memory as an aid to alleviating and preventing problems. It is like the continental road signs: primitive, vivid and direct. It compels action. The 'Nurse in a Tizzy' is perhaps easy to spot, but the cartoon signposts the message: Danger! Stop! How can I help? with such clarity that it can hardly be forgotten. Cartoons are outrageous—and by halting reality may re-route our ideas.

'Please act quickly!'

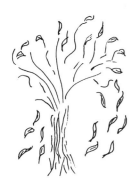

Nothing could more vividly illustrate the feelings of the junior member of the team who has blundered and been reprimanded by her seniors beyond endurance than the withered tree—a brilliant piece of empathy on the part of one of her seniors who courageously brought her own incident to a group. 'Is *this* what we're doing to our juniors!' a nursing officer said in dismay. This piece of shorthand, this signposting action, is unlikely to be forgotten: the emotion is too powerful to be ignored. Little touches, acute observation matter: the tall, empty house has a mat with 'Welcome' on it: but the sick man is alone with his cat, and no one is there to supervise his diet. . . . Nurse, doctor, and social worker are unlikely to forget the dangers of failing to coordinate, with this *aide memoire* imprinted on their minds.

In another drawing the client was first expressed as a rather dim and inactive

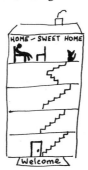

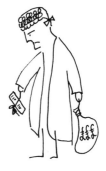

pin man, without even a mouth to speak with. At a later stage the drawing suggested in a single glance the need for the team to work closely together in support of the hapless nurse who was now seen to be in the clutches of a litigating relative. Problem and action became clearer.

'What am I?'

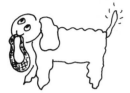

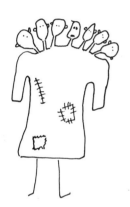

Another change of drawing from the straightforward to the Walt Disney dream world is more than startling: it shows the relationship between a speech therapy student and her superior in a way that suggested to them both some of their immediate problems. For the student doing the drawings, this was the first time she had realized her difficulties—and in a way which indicated action. She, for instance, while gazing in adoration at her senior and bringing her little gifts, might do well to prepare herself for her own future. A future in which she will appear like Cinderella, overworked and underpaid; in her turn, doing not only speech therapy, but the chores of seven other people. Moreover, seven heads are drawn, but there is only one mouth to speak with! Will she, when she becomes a senior, lack the voice to make her professional needs known, the arms to reach out to *her* clients, *her* colleagues, *her* juniors?

'What am I?' said student and her supervisor, as they analysed the incident together. In this case, the senior immediately broadened the training of her student to include management politics, a lesson not lost upon other disciplines observing the session.

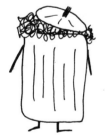

The conscious honesty of a young ward sister as she drew herself as she imagined others—especially her seniors—saw her, led to even deeper questioning. In the thick of a battle between the training school's idea of cleanliness, tidiness and perfection and the reality of her ward as it is on a busy day, this cartoon led the group to point out to her that this same battle is raged inside each individual nurse and that she was not alone in asking herself: 'What am I—a nurse or a skivvy? A cleaner—or a comforter? A dustbin!'

'It really isn't done to show your feelings!'

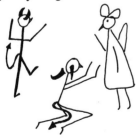

Details drawn unconsciously often reveal deeply felt attitudes which purely verbal discussion is unlikely to bring out. It is simply not done, for instance, to hate a patient. The image of a nurse as an angel of mercy, often drawn as a pin man with a halo, is an image not normally connected with feelings of resentment and anger. But nurses are human, the feelings may be there—sometimes, with some patients. The fury expressed here by drawing the patient as the first Devil was probably only surpassed by the sweet revenge of the second—for whoever saw the Devil with horns drooping and his tail between his legs! But that nurse said he felt the bitterness drain away as he drew.

32

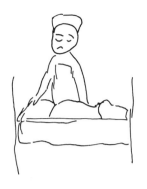

Place a whip in the hands of bullying relatives (as in the Four Sons) and you and the group have faced together some highly unacceptable feelings. The cartoon *allows* you to feel, it is socially acceptable to express anger and hatred and bitterness in this joking fashion; and so the guilt attached to them is likely to fade. The despair and the grief when a sick baby dies, the slump of the shoulders as the nurse stands by the bed reveal feelings normally covered up by a brisk efficiency. This drawing was almost a throw-away, a sideline to the main incident: the feeling in the simple lines is, however, intense.

'I daren't say so, but—'

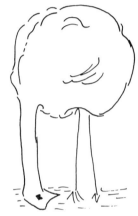

The spontaneous grin of delight when one group suddenly realized that they could suspend reality and draw as they really felt, suggested in itself the tension behind the story. Illustrating the doctor as an ostrich, head in the sand, released much of this tension. Similarly, cartooning the psychiatrist as an amiable, well-meaning donkey, not giving much support in the nurses' eyes, released much of the bitterness by the very act of analysing and capturing this aspect of the medical team.

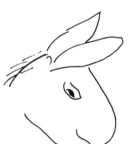

Drawing has two benefits: Firstly concentration is needed to decide whom to put in the picture, how and where to draw them, which details it is essential to portray, and in what order and what size—such concentration will in itself reduce the more negative emotions and anxieties. Secondly, when drawings are in the form of cartoons, the group relaxes in discussing what object or animal, what lines, what angles will best express how they feel about one of their characters. Their efforts at drawing these exaggerated pictures and the humorous appreciation of other groups, releases tension, anger and bitterness where words might well have reinforced all three.

Few of the incidents and even fewer of the constructive ideas emerging from discussion are likely to be remembered in the pressures of everyday work. Consider how much those who have been on courses actually remember and use the information they have absorbed? But a dramatic cartoon-style drawing, because of its humour and exaggeration, is likely to flash through the mind when another similar situation occurs. The Wobbly Jelly . . . the Withered Tree . . . the Nurse in a Tizzy . . . can *you* forget them?

Don't talk—draw!

Part 2—Hidden depths

4. Whither communication?

Objectives to the chapter

1. To analyse through three Illuminative Incidents various facets of communication, moving from the more obvious, overt problems to the hidden, covert attitudes and perceptions.

2. To develop awareness of some of the mischievous blocks which render the term irrelevant.

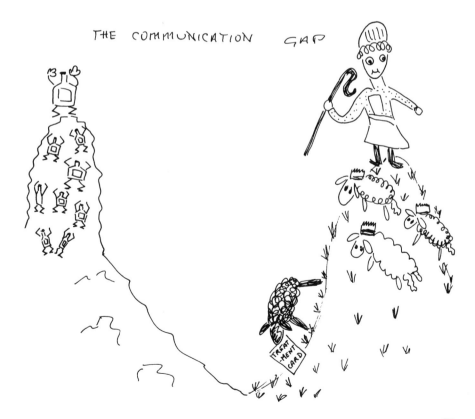

THE COMMUNICATION GAP

Where do we go from here?

Just as it is important for the traveller that the guide book should differentiate between Cambridge, England and Cambridge, Massachussets: similarly for the nurse, it is important that someone should differentiate between two Mrs Smiths in the same ward. Failure in either situation, is likely to cause confusion; confusion which will be imputed to lack of communication. But is this the whole story?

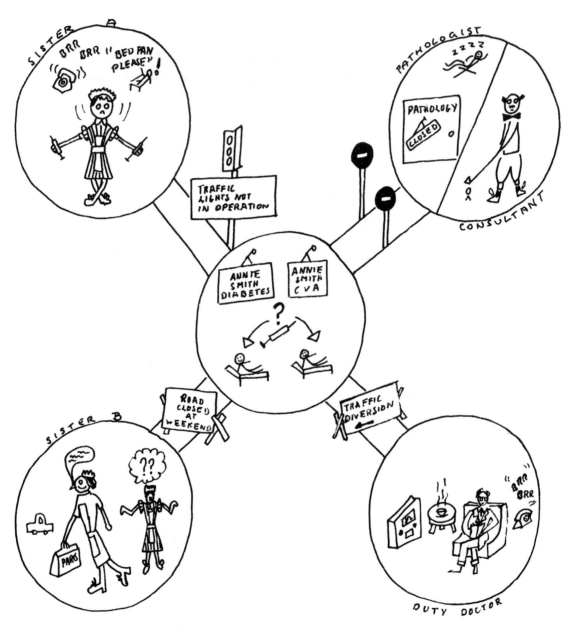

The name's the same—Who's to blame!

Incident: *two Mrs Annie Smiths were given each other's treatment and both suffered in consequence.*

There were two Mrs Annie Smiths on Hyacinth Ward, both recovering happily: one was a heart case and the other a diabetic. Sister A had successfully sorted out which was which before she went off duty. Sister B needed to change their beds round—and told everyone on duty she had done so.

Hand-over time next day was busy, noisy and confused, and Sister B was rushing off for a much-needed holiday. Forgetting she hadn't told Sister A about the changed beds, she left to catch her plane. In fact, everyone who knew about the two Mrs Annie Smiths, assumed that Sister A knew, and acted accordingly.

Too late, Sister A discovered the change: the Mrs Smiths had already been given each other's treatment.

Consultant and pathologist, relaxing over the weekend, were not available to help sort out the muddle and there were serious consequences for both Mrs Smiths.

In their drawing the group chose a street scene to illustrate the overt problems they saw, with the helpless Mrs Smiths cut off from everyone, and the team itself isolated by the events of the weekend.

The first questions, inevitably, were: would the incident have been averted if clear, typed memos had been placed on sister's desk; if similar surnames on the ward had been typed in red; if all off-duty staff had been at the end of a telephone . . . the group, drawing their road-blocks, decided not. There was more to the problem than this.

In addition to the conflicting calls upon her of: Telephone! (administration) and: Bedpan! (patient care) the bewildered nurse is burdened with incomprehensible instructions—for *which* Mrs Annie Smith? Sister B, off for a jaunty weekend, is too full of dreams to remember every tiny detail at hand-over time. Pathologist, consultant, registrar—they too, have other things on their minds. Perhaps *they* know which Mrs Smith is which . . . or do they?

One thing is certain: everything that should have been done, was done properly; every routine instruction had been followed; it was a good ward, in a first-class hospital. And yet the mistake happened, with serious consequences.

Exploration of road blocks

The first group had time only to realize that they needed to study in depth the reasons why all the roads were blocked simultaneously, aware that there were other factors behind the lack of communication, they had no opportunity to explore them. In the next incident, Peter's Leg, one of the authors—partially responsible for the tragedy—had time, motivation and opportunity for delving beneath the surface to the deeper, covert reasons behind the so-called lack of communication.

Incident: *a mentally handicapped man was run over and his leg was severely injured.*

Peter, a young, bright, adult resident in a hospital for the mentally handicapped, asked the doctor if he could have a job outside the hospital. The social worker found him employment the other side of the local town and took him to the interview in her car.

Six members of staff knew from gossip, or suspected that Peter had never crossed a road alone in his life, but they said nothing. The author realizing the situation and having, as organizer of voluntary workers, the means of providing training in road safety, met the social worker on a corridor the day before Peter started his new job. They chatted about him. But—'Why should *I* tell her about Peter,' the author thought to herself, 'silly old duck! Let her find out for herself. It's not my job!' She said nothing.

Peter was run over on his way to work, badly injuring his leg, and was unable to walk for six months.

The author explored this as a straight communication problem: who had spoken to whom? This is the first diagram: Diagram of Communication (below). It presents a vivid picture, alarming enough, of an almost totally non-communicating team. It did not, however, in any way explain why several staff in a caring profession had said nothing to any of their colleagues about Peter's inability to cross the road.

The second diagram, Map of Communication, was in the form of a flow-chart, showing in a simple map, who went where and who spoke to whom. It revealed the two moments at which the accident might have been prevented, *if . . . if* the doctor had made a round of the Occupation Department where Peter worked, she could have met either the psychologist and asked for a report on Peter, or the voluntary work organizer and asked for a road safety check. Similarly, on her ward round, she could have asked the nurse to do this. *If*, later on, the social worker had trodden the same path, she too might have prevented the accident . . . or so it seemed.

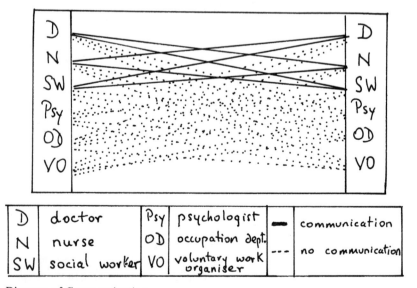

Diagram of Communication

The Map of Communication showed a lot: the physical separation of ward and occupation unit, the isolation of all the members of the team, the ignorance of both doctor and social worker about the roles of those able to provide information—had they been asked. But it still did not really solve the deeper problem: why did the author, a senior, responsible, caring professional feel about one of her patients: 'It's not my business', and about one of her hard-working colleagues: 'Let her find out for herself'?

The Picture of Communication sums up the basic, covert situation and it becomes evident that there are many flash points.

The customary leader, the doctor, is faceless and unknown: not seen as giving any kind of support or leadership. Nor is the social worker, though a larger figure, seen in a leadership role—nor even linked with a team. The barred, invisible occupation unit hardly invites cooperation, and certainly would deter any visitor; and the devil figure is one with which we are familiar by

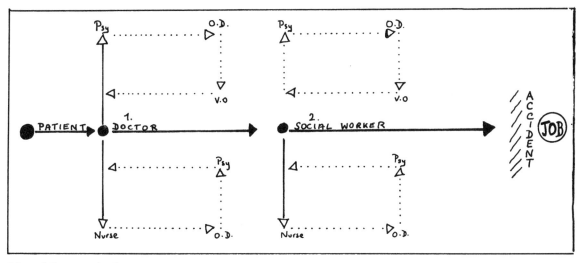

Map of Communication

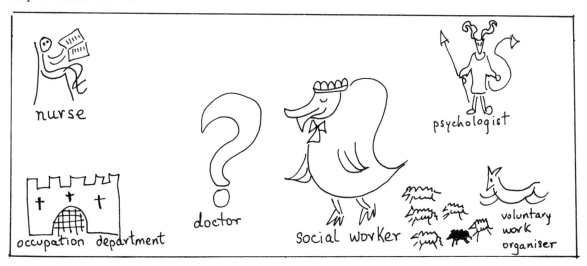

Picture of Communication

now, and likely to avoid where possible. One has only to add an apathetic nurse and an irrelevantly energetic voluntary organizer, chasing up everyone except herself, to see that something was bound to flare up. Who was the leader—and where was the team? And who was supporting whom?

In the world of mental handicap—not the easiest of jobs, emotionally—to be faced with additional emotional problems in a disintegrated team as this, is an almost intolerable burden. Peter was the one to suffer.

Since Illuminative Incident Analysis is a constructive technique, positive action did result from Peter's Leg. It is described in chapter 7.

From two people with the same name, an example revealing fairly obvious blocked channels of communication, to examples of some covert blocks: these incidents show clear indications of the immediate problems. For a deeper look at the emotional aspects—those dangerous, hidden nine-tenths of the iceberg which do the damage, we look at an incident which a different group was able to analyse in depth. They started where the others left off, and tried to penetrate the hidden mainsprings of communication: motives, attitudes, perceptions. It was a group with an unusually wide range of hospital, education and local authority staff who, together with four visitors, analysed the incident. The fact that many of the group were strangers both to each other and to the hospital may possibly account for the depths covered in one morning.

'I Want to be Loved'

Incident: *Charlie smashes several windows on the ward.*
Charlie, a cheeky little boy living in a hospital for the mentally handi-capped, goes every day to the school which stands in the hospital grounds. The teachers there are not employed by the hospital, but come under the local education authority. One Friday afternoon, Charlie is told by his teacher that he is going home with his parents for the weekend and he gets very excited.

When he gets back to his ward at teatime, the overworked—and perhaps better informed—nurse tells him curtly that his parents are *not* coming for him that weekend, that he is *not* going home.

Competing disciplines

SCHOOL
Laissez-faire

"He's Improving!"

WARD
Authoritarian

"He's deteriorating!"

Halos and horns depicted the sheer emotion of the group's first reaction. But the signs are the same for Charlie as they were for the two Mrs Smiths: all roads communicating between them and the staff around them were blocked. In stark terms of black-and-white, good-and-evil, the two competing disciplines of teaching and nursing are making dramatically opposed statements about both themselves and Charlie. *Their attitude* to the boy is conflicting; *their judgement* of the boy is completely different; *their perception* of each other is uncompromising, different—and dangerous. No one, given these three factors, is likely to listen, let alone to communicate. (And it is sometimes forgotten that listening is as vital as talking.) Charlie is doomed from the start. Each side has forgotten him. Each is concentrating upon using the natural physical and professional distance between school and ward to main-tain warfare and (as one of the group whose story this was, confessed) to prevent communication. But all these attitudes become clear only when drawing and commenting on the Angels and Devils.

42

Brick wall

Illuminative Incident Analysis is rather like peeling an onion: there is always a further layer to remove—and the deeper the layer, the more copious the tears! 'The purpose of making anything,' says the sculptor Reg Butler, 'is to discover what it is going to be . . . The sense of seeing where one is going, is after one has gone.' So it is with the more rewarding explorations of Illuminative Incidents.

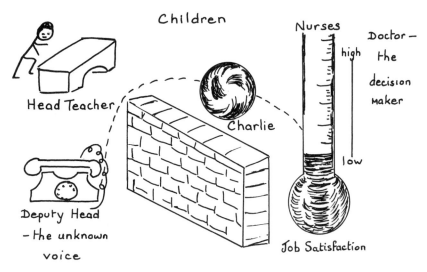

Brick wall and ping-pong ball

The important feature at the start of this second drawing was the brick wall. But this time, the group decided to put themselves on the side of the Devils, and draw things from Satan's point of view: a highly practical exercise in role perception and an example of a group organizing its own learning process.

Having done this, the group began to see where they were going—and they did not like it. On the one side of the solid brick wall they had illustrated themselves (the Devils) as a depersonalized thermometer: this, in a supposedly warm situation which was Charlie's second home, with the nurses in the role of substitute parents. In addition the thermometer registered low job satisfaction. On the other side was the head teacher, who had never been known to communicate with the nurses nor give a report on the children's progress. Beneath her was a deputy head who made communicating noises over the telephone. But she did not really respond to the need the nurses said they had for face-to-face discussion on methods of handling the children: a common situation.

Ping-pong ball

It was when someone inserted Charlie in the form of a ping-pong ball spinning from one side of the wall to the other, that the group really began to realize what they had drawn. The sequence of frustration-to-apathy was clearer now. The group was now able to observe that apathy, masking the energetic anger of the battle between Angels and Devils, was causing this energy to be diverted to bat and slice Charlie from one side of the wall to the other. The whole conference was shocked by this vivid depiction of a child being used in this way by two separate, professional teams. Game or battle, the situation was readily recognized by many in the audience, whatever their job, and several left the session determined to take action to search out and help the 'ping-pong ball clients' in their own organizations.

'I want to be loved by both sides!'

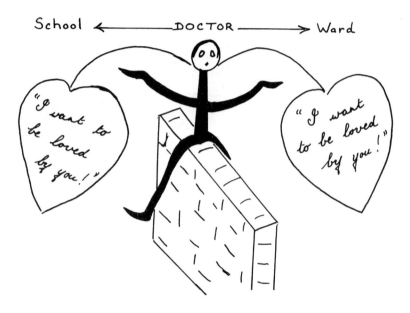

This simpler, final drawing explored the missing figure: the doctor, a psychiatrist. He had first been drawn as just a label in a corner of the paper on the side of the Devils—the side with low job satisfaction. At last, the crucial question: Why the battle? could be answered. Over a coffee break, the group suddenly realized that, far from being on the edge of things, he was right in the centre of the game, the key figure. His inability to take decisions and lead the team had puzzled them, until this was seen as perhaps a desire to please both sides: a style of leadership certain to bring insecurity. The team is not being led: it is actually being *divided* by the accepted leader, the doctor.

It is interesting to speculate here: why, when the group discovered attitudes in themselves that they did not like, did they continue the uncomfortable process of exploration?

We do not pretend that self-discovery is ever an easy process. At a surface level, Illuminative Incident Analysis has been described as a rather jolly way of looking at what is happening; it may teach staff or students to consider roles, job satisfaction, priorities—and many other facets which can become almost academic, even in the realistic, operational setting of ward or unit. But exploring in depth has something in common with the 'Ulysses' factor: a restless urge to find out, an urge to do something difficult, to know oneself, perhaps to prove oneself. It is this deep curiosity which seems almost

irresistible to those who painfully search beneath the surface, and in searching change their attitudes both to colleagues and to their work. This, it is to be
presumed, is their reward—and the impetus to further exploration. It is this
'Ulysses' mechanism which makes Illuminative Incident Analysis a dynamic
technique for those with the courage to learn about themselves.

Exit communication

Procedures, memos, telephone messages—these are all facets of communication.
But these were not the root causes of Charlie's miserable protest. He was
merely reflecting the deeper problems of relationships, of apathy, of well-
meaning but weak leadership; all of which were blocking the channels of
communication. And if communication is not, as it at first appeared, the
basic factor in this breakdown of service to a client, if it is attitudes, perceptions, motives that are unhealthy, the team will be sick, no matter how
firm is the prescription—'Get Talking'.

> 'Didn't anyone send a memo?'
> 'Did you leave a 'phone message?'
> 'Why didn't someone tell me that?'

We assume that to communicate people should be sending notes and using
the 'phone. If we don't know a thing, we assume it is because they didn't
tell us. But memos get put in the waste-paper basket—or filed in a dusty
drawer; people give you messages when your diary is not in your hand; and
the telephone rings when you're talking to someone. Even if you receive the
memo or phone call, you interpret what the other person says in *your* terms—
which may be quite a different thing.

Of memos it has been said:

> 'This place is just teeming with memos. We send them to every conceivable
> person, it takes up a lot of time, but coordination isn't good at all.'

Coordination, Communication, Cooperation—the 'Big Cs', the in-terms of the
'seventies:

> 'Coordination is a term seldom defined. A team is
> formed, a conference held, a report written and sent.
> Coordination: an arranging, an organising, a system-
> atising process, has taken place. So too has com-
> munication: a sharing, a diffusing, a disseminating
> of knowledge. But labelling a group of professionals
> 'a team' is to confuse idea with action. Holding a
> conference does not necessarily result in working to-
> gether. Writing a report in no way ensures either the
> intelligent reading of it or action upon it.'*

There is evidently more to communication than creating a team, issuing
orders, devising a routine, agreeing an emergency procedure. If a team solves
its other problems: those of working together constructively, of attitudes
and perceptions of each other's roles, for instance, then communication takes

* *Action Learning, 1972.* A King Edward's Hospital Fund Publication,
London.

care of itself and the term becomes unnecessary. But if a team is *unhealthy*, the term becomes a red herring which hinders effective team development. And the beguiling diagrams, charts and lists that flower on office walls after any reorganization will remain after the first fine rapture as just a talking point for visitors.

Communication is spoken of in capital letters and awed voice as if it were the main problem: but if a team is healthy in other respects then communication as a problem in itself ceases to exist.

'Have meetings—will talk!'
Do *you* think 'communication'
is the universal panacea?

5. Follow my leader

Objectives to the chapter

1. To look at leadership problems.
2. To discover neglected members of the team
3. To find the patient.

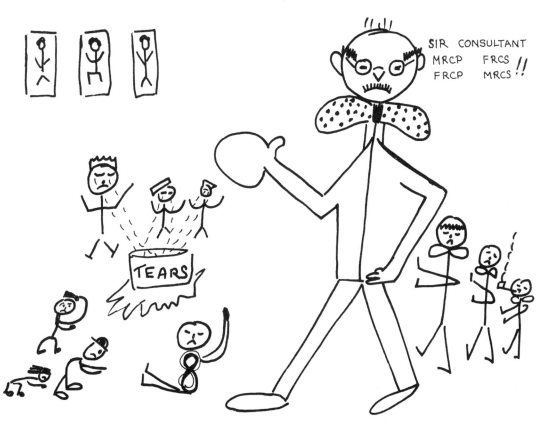

While one may, in modern management, question the necessity for a leader, or at least for a permanent leader, problems do arise when a team expects leadership of a traditional kind and does not get it. In the cartoons we have so far found seven types of uneasy leadership which contribute to a sick or maladjusted team.

Leadership

The Big White Chief
(or: The God Syndrome)

Dominant leadership, so feelingly illustrated here, brings more than one problem, for not only do the domineered tend in their turn to dominate the next one down and so destroy the sense of teamwork, but the Big White Chief with appalling frequency sees no need to commune with those in the ranks.

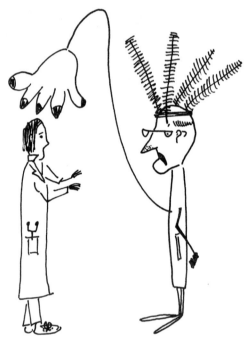

Big White Chief

Not surprisingly, the Big White Chief is paralleled by the Lady Chieftain. Like the consultant, she too dominates her juniors. But she angrily stamps her foot and gets 'steamed-up'. With the Lady Chieftain, however, it is for a real misdemeanour and results in a more submissive junior. Whereas the Big White Chief is illustrated as dominant because he himself feels superior, and his lofty air produces a limp junior in attendance, the Lady Chieftain is always drawn as more emotional, with a frightened junior at her feet.

One incident showed how difficult it was for a nurse when neither she nor the registrar had been told by the surgeon just how serious an apparently simple operation was. They therefore had no idea that symptoms which could safely be ignored in most cases, in this particular case were indicative of danger. No one was prepared to question 'God', and it was instinct, experience or luck, said the nurse, that kept the patient alive.

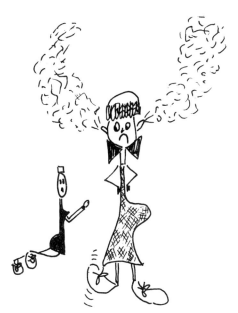

Lady Chieftain

It is an extremely difficult feat to put yourself in the shoes of 'God'. But perceptively some of our groups have been able to draw incidents from the viewpoint of the Big White Chief, and, in so doing, have come to realize how much some of these difficult people need support in their own insecurity. They have also seen through their drawings, that 'God' can be human, and that they might have the courage to approach him.

> **Incident**: *A patient who happened to be a consultant, sick in his own hospital, cancelled an ambulance ordered for another patient.*
> The consultant, uneasily a patient on his own ward, sits in bed, cantankerous, demanding: one eye on the clock—insisting on treatment on the dot, stethoscope at the ready to check, one hand imperiously waving all junior staff away. He was the most troublesome patient, issuing orders from his private room—he was loathed.

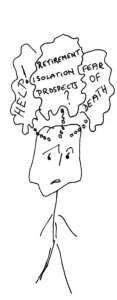

> Finally deigning to talk to another patient, the consultant learns that this man is to be sent home by ambulance. 'Not necessary!' he decrees, 'You can go by private car through the Red Cross.' And he immediately 'phones the transport office and cancels the ambulance, causing much confusion to office and ward and patient.

Encouraged to delve beneath the rigid surface he presented, the nurses found themselves drawing this picture of a depressed, sad and insecure old man. They had suddenly seen a human being behind the status of the role.

Although this is not a solution to the God syndrome, it does offer one explanation which must surely be acceptable, and in this case it certainly softened the nurses' feelings. Their attitude to difficult seniors would in future be more tolerant, they said. Such understanding might in turn give the Big White Chief more support and so perhaps less need to be domineering. It may not be possible to change his personality—but it may make him easier to work with.

But the God Syndrome can exist at all levels and the hall porter, the receptionist, the telephonist—not usually seen as leaders, nor even as part of the team, may still play the game. They, too, can withhold information with results every bit as disastrous for the patient as when the consultant does it. They, too, can take decisions which affect the client. It was the hall porter who, knowing that the ambulance was not due to fetch a very sick patient for transfer to another hospital until late afternoon, watched that patient propped up with increasing discomfort in a wheelchair from nine o'clock in the morning. 'Not *my* job to tell anyone!' he decided.

Divided leadership

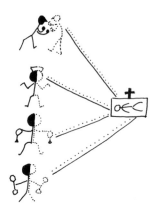

Incident: *a patient died while the treatment team were quarrelling.*
Two consultants fell out and the fight between them became public knowledge. It was in an overseas hospital and they shared nursing staff, registrars and technicians on the ward. The rest of the team felt forced to take sides and from the top down were split in two, each side obeying the orders of its own leader. Neither consultant would agree whose responsibility it was to order blood for a patient, and because the team followed suit, the patient died untreated while waiting for the argument to be settled.

This incident dramatically illustrated by the group, who coloured each person half red and half green, provoked considerable discussion on the consequences of irresponsible leadership seen in men who are highly qualified in their own specialty, but ignorant of the skills of managing the team.

The group containing one of the doctors concerned, suggested a delightful solution: place red and green bundles on the conference table, the one representing all the negative causes of the incident, the other, the team's strengths and assets. 'Build constructively with the green bundles!' they cried—and went away with every intention of doing so themselves.

Anonymous leaderships: 'They'

The God Syndrome is usually an obvious affair and 'God' can usually be pinpointed. 'They' is a phenomenon closely linked in many respects, and familiar to us all: but who are 'They'? 'They' seldom are drawn.

The flower bed
Incident: *old people were not allowed to have a flower bed that was planned for them.*
An old peoples' unit had a beautiful view of a pond with ducks, and willow trees around it. Then a workshop, a grey concrete slab building, was erected on a piece of spare ground—entirely obscuring the view of the pond.

The ward sister used initiative, and arranged for a group of volunteers to dig and plant some flower beds in front of the unit for the old people to look at. The volunteers bought spades, forks and plants and agreed on a rota to maintain the beds. At this point, the scheme was mysteriously vetoed from above by 'Them'. It was not hospital policy to have flower beds, the sister was told.

This is a delightfully typical 'They' incident: a decision taken by remote control, incomprehensible, irreversible. It leaves its victims helpless. 'They', is perhaps one of the biggest enemies of dynamic development in any organization. And yet, from the very fact that we have no cartoons of 'They', only one or two vague attempts at drawing a faceless committee sitting round an endless table, it is obvious that one of the problems is inability to identify this mystical force which seems always to be working against us. We, of course, are never 'They'.

The new leader

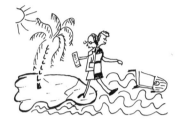

The two-headed, recently promoted nurse administrator illustrated here shows her dilemma: when faced with a fumbling junior, does she herself supervise the patient's treatment as only she knows how? Or does she, like the well-trained administrator she has now become, just 'delegate downwards' and retire to the palmy shores of office life? We are all faced at times with the undeniable fact that it is often quicker and easier to do a thing ourselves; the misfortune of the senior nurse is that so often it is a question of life or death.

Patient as leader

A young ward sister illustrated, with devastating honesty, her realization of what happened to her team when she herself was working with one eye on the promotion ladder (see page 52).

Queen Bee
Incident: *a teenage girl in a general hospital took a second overdose after an argument with another patient.*
Tracy was a tearaway teenager with elderly parents. After treatment for an overdose of drugs, she was sent to recuperate in a ward which dealt with elderly ladies suffering from heart disease. Tracy's world was that of noisy pop music and none-too-clean, torn jeans; as she recovered, remaining in the hospital for psychiatric treatment, she found herself in a world of quiet but cantankerous sick women.

Apparently now fit and merely 'a nuisance to everyone', Tracy was found one evening in bed, unconscious from a second overdose of drugs.

These nurses, one of the first groups to discover the depths to which they could probe a situation through the use of cartoons, eventually saw what had gone wrong: one of the elderly patients was running the ward—the domineering Queen Bee. The young ward sister, shut up inside her anthill as she busily builds it higher and higher towards promotion, seems unaware that she is virtually cut off from both her staff and her patients, with no idea (until the drawing was done) that Tracy is isolated, too.

The ward sister who was involved in this incident was shaken by her discovery, and by the end of the session was actively planning to make stronger links with her nurses and more contact with her patients.

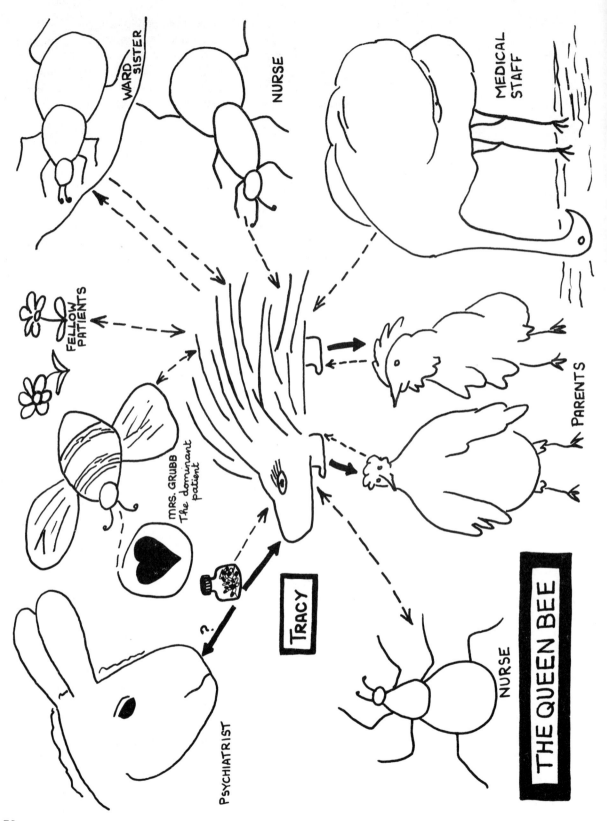

WARD SISTER

NURSE

MEDICAL STAFF

FELLOW PATIENTS

PARENTS

MRS. GRUBB
The dominant patient

?

PSYCHIATRIST

TRACY

NURSE

THE QUEEN BEE

In a different setting, the problem of leadership was revealed in a local authority department combining social services, medical services and housing.

In common with the ward sister in the Queen Bee, the person concerned in this incident (who analysed it alone) discovered as she drew her cartoon that although she had the impression she was in close contact with a wide number of colleagues across the social and local government services she was in reality, quite cut off. After looking at her own drawing which is shown on page 54, she, too, took active steps to remedy the situation.

Florrie

Incident: *an old lady was found alone in her flat, surrounded by luggage and in tears. She had been crying for four hours.*

Florrie, aged eighty, was sent by a housing officer from her flat in one old people's home, to another home across the town, while her own flat was being decorated.

It so happened that during this period the only person available to act as night duty standby in Florrie's original home was this same housing officer. As a personal favour, she agreed to sleep in the warden's flat while the warden was on leave, with her permission. Inadvertently, the warden's maid put out a favourite tablecloth for breakfast, and when the warden discovered this on returning from her holiday, she took it as a deliberate affront on the part of the housing officer, and ceased to communicate with her from that moment.

So, when Florrie's flat was ready and she was due to return from her temporary home, the warden's anger against the housing officer took the form of 'paying her out'—by not informing her (or anyone else) of Florrie's movements. Florrie therefore arrived back quite alone, without the social worker, the housing officer—or the warden—to a newly-decorated room which, in her confusion, she failed to recognize as her own. There was no one to reassure her, or to help her unpack, and she was found some hours later still in her outdoor clothes, suitcases by her side, standing in tears.

This is an almost unbelievable example of paying someone out for an imagined slight, a process several of our groups have labelled 'tit-for-tattery.' We discuss it further in the next chapter.

Here, it illustrates to a remarkable degree the isolation of all four main characters: the two wardens, the social worker and the housing officer. It appears that none of them considered that there was either team or leader. The housing officer, since she had close connections with the old people's homes and with the social services, *thought* she was leading when she made arrangements by telephone and left messages. Clearly, the others did not see her as a leader . . . nor was she herself quite clear if this was her role.

In the confusion, poor Florrie is pushed to one side of the drawing, the isolated position in which the client is often found where an incident occurs. And only during the actual act of drawing, was it realized that the social worker was on a bicycle. Had he had a car, the incident just might have been averted, since he personally, could have brought Florrie back home.

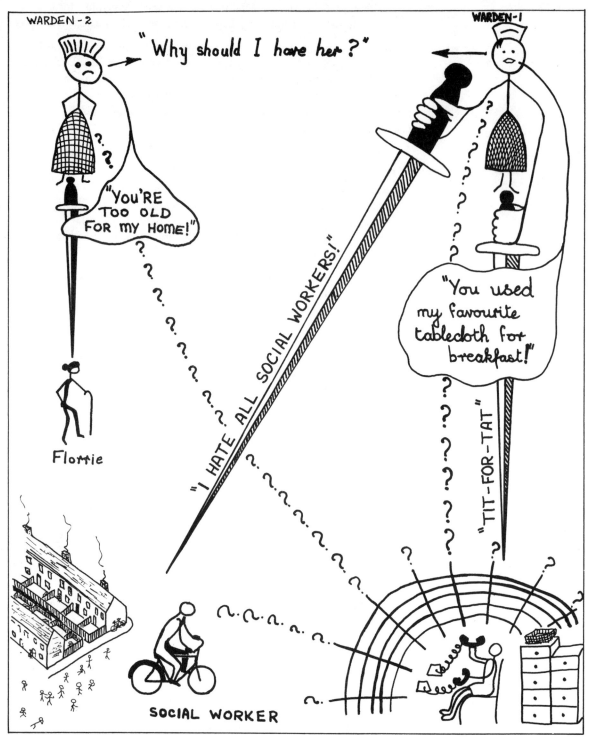

"FLORRIE"

A constructive result, during the years that followed the analysis of this incident, was that the housing officer, who was appalled at what she had learned about herself and her department, took active steps to ensure clear communication. Realizing now some of the problems that lie behind *communication*, she has ensured that there is a supportive team with informed and involved juniors who are also made aware of the pitfalls.

Anarchy

Finally, in the problems of leadership, we reach the ultimate chaos of: Who leads? Do I lead? Aren't you the leader? This illustration came from one of the overseas doctors working on the incident described in the section on Divided Leadership. After the red-green drawings, showing the team split by two warring consultants, this drawing suggests the ultimate stage of allowing such a battle to continue: anarchy in the jungle . . . the jungle beasts at war . . . the storm clouds rolling above the tangled trees. Interestingly, this illustration started as a cannon, a weapon of conventional warfare; as the doctor drawing it relaxed and really 'drew from his stomach', suspending reality, this nightmare of a leaderless, divided team emerged, and shocked all who saw the drawing.

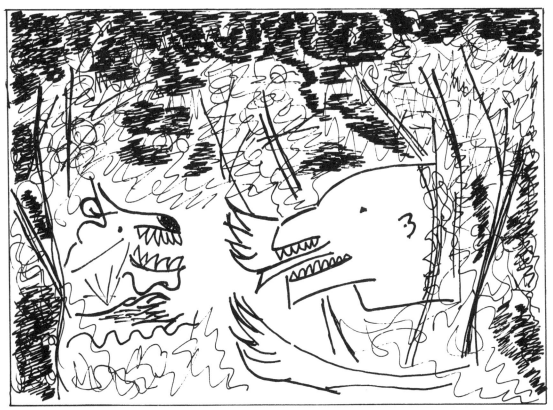

Jungle warfare

Look at **your** *leadership*

Problems in leadership may seem easy to identify: the difficulty often lies in persuading the leader to see an incident as anything other than incompetence on the part of his juniors, or as some failure in technology or procedure. It is evidently only the secure and flexible leader who can really listen to his team, or even encourage his team to speak freely about their problems. Nonetheless, there are many like the young ward sister in Queen Bee, who can with honesty and humour, draw an incident, stop in their tracks and say: 'Good heavens! Is this what I am? How can I change?'

What we do not know, as yet, is how to persuade the less flexible or adventurous, to see themselves from the outside, as others see them. However gently done, with however much sympathy and humour, it is never a comfortable process, for any of us.

We cannot expect dramatic changes overnight, and it is not our role as tutor to offer solutions to other people's problems. But our groups suggested questions which we could all ask ourselves, either as leaders or followers—for every leader among us is, in some situations, himself a follower.

▶ I have a Big White Chief. . . . How am I in turn treating *my* juniors?
▶ I *am* a Big White Chief. . . . Do I really talk to people?
▶ Do I communicate with my leader?
▶ How can I help my leader?
▶ Do I talk about 'They'? Am I ever one of 'Them' myself?
▶ Where are the new leaders in my world and how can I support them?
▶ Who leads my team? Who thinks I do?
▶ Do I ever catch myself thinking: 'My juniors are incompetent'—or do I try to learn from them?
▶ How often do I talk about: shortages
　　　　　　　　　　　　　　: failures in technology
　　　　　　　　　　　　　　: lack of defined procedures?

Who follows?

It is not the place of this book to consider the broader principles of teams in the whole range of health and social services, of hospital and community staff. Who is in a team is often obvious, but we are pursuing still the hidden nine-tenths of the iceberg, the concealed strengths of a team. We are also concerned to report through the eyes of our groups *their* world as *they* see it through exploring *their* incidents. Here, then, we bring together individuals who are often overlooked, proposing them—as did the groups concerned—for full team membership.

Relatives

The Champion
Incident: *none of the staff realized that a man was on steroids, and in consequence, after a relatively simple hernia operation he was seriously ill.*
The patient's wife, the Champion, made sure that his own doctor wrote about the steroids to the surgeon; she told all the nurses she could find, and the registrar. Despite her heroic efforts to inform everyone, nobody took any notice: she was 'a bit of a nuisance' to busy staff, always going on and on about her husband. Without steroids his life was endangered, and, indeed, at one stage after the operation his pulse and respiration

indicated serious trouble. Fortunately for the patient, the medical students listened to his wife and steroids were administered eventually.

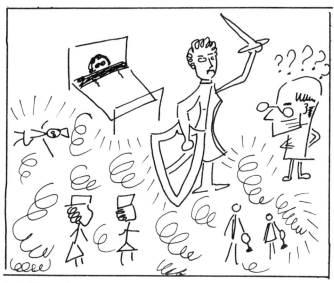

The Champion

The Champion fought tirelessly, but was ignored until it was almost too late. She is illustrated defending her husband, who lies bewildered by the confusion around him. She is, in effect, part of that team.

Stella, another wife, was invited to join her husband's team as an active outcome of Illuminative Incident Analysis. She participated fully in the design of the treatment programme for her husband. She was lucky. 'How can we on the staff best help you?' she was asked at a case conference. Startled, she was silent, but wrote the next day: 'I was unable to answer because I'd never thought of you as helping *me* . . . You've always been 'Them', and I've always been fighting you!'

The vigour and energy of these wives, however misplaced it may seem to the staff—and of the Four Sons whose negative strivings on behalf of their mother, that caused such distress to a ward sister—is a bonus that no team concerned with caring for its clients can afford to waste.

Cinderellas

'Don't sweep your dirt under the carpet!' we are saying, 'It contains valuable treasure for building your team successfully.' So, in the allegorical world of cartoons developed by our groups, it is not surprising that we should find Cinderella. Hard-working, indispensable, hidden from sight and sometimes ill-rewarded, our Cinderellas in the social services are not by any means necessarily in 'menial' jobs. But one thing they do have in common: their work is unglamorous and seldom attracts the limelight. One might even find a senior Cinderella such as a consultant in an unpopular or chronic specialty.

From a long list of Cinderellas: porters, ambulance men, pharmacists, laboratory technicians, telephonists, radiographers . . . we pick a story not only concerned with, but analysed *by* a group of Cinderellas in a subnormality hospital—student nurses.

This was a group containing many overseas students, some with language problems and all preoccupied with working hard to pass exams. The incident is another trivial, commonplace one which was explored over four sessions. At first the class was not over-enthusiastic, perhaps because they were used to being taught a specific, orthodox topic and found this learning method strange. Certainly they found it a difficult exercise initially.

Broken Promises

Incident: *Jane hit and bit the staff and broke a window.*
Jane, a young and troublesome adolescent in a long-stay hospital, found out that there was a coach trip to the seaside that very afternoon. Jane had 'a thing' about coach trips, always clamouring to join the party, but—because she is so difficult to control—was never allowed to.

Somehow or other, Jane contrived to be beside the coach as it picked up its passengers, and she stood shouting louder and louder: 'I want to go, I want to go, I want to go!' Alice, a student nurse, calmed her down with great difficulty, firmly repeating: 'No—you cannot go on the coach today, it's *not* your turn,'—when a middle-aged play leader passed by.

The play leader was a soft-hearted lady, new to the hospital world. 'There, Jane' she said, 'of course you can go on the coach if you want to.' But the outing was, in any case, for the children only.

Jane's yells crescendoed as the coach drove off, and she bit and hit everyone who came near her, finally smashing a window.

The first drawing confirmed the suspicion that there were just two ways of dealing with the continually difficult and demanding Jane. They illustrated this, more with words than drawings:

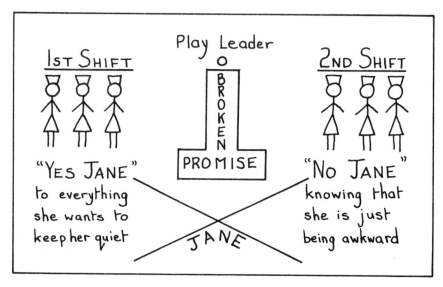

'Yes Jane—No Jane!'

'We've finished!' announced the students, 'it's just a matter of organizing ward meetings and *making* the two shifts communicate.'

It is to the credit of the group that, after a lot of circular discussion on these lines, they did finally settle down to explore in a more relaxed style—but only after the tutor firmly pointed out that regular meetings were held on the ward already.

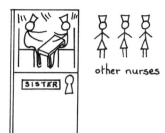

other nurses

Immediately, it became apparent to the students that the lack of communication was a puzzle, since all the ward staff concerned with Jane worked from nine to five, except the ward sisters, who had a hand-over session at lunch-time . . . but what did the two ward sisters say to each other? No one knew.

So who was really involved with Jane, and who really spoke to whom? The next diagram explored this.

A very different problem now emerged from that first posed by the incident. People *were* communicating, but not throughout the complete team. In fact there were two teams, 'Yes Jane' and 'No Jane'. Those who talked to young,

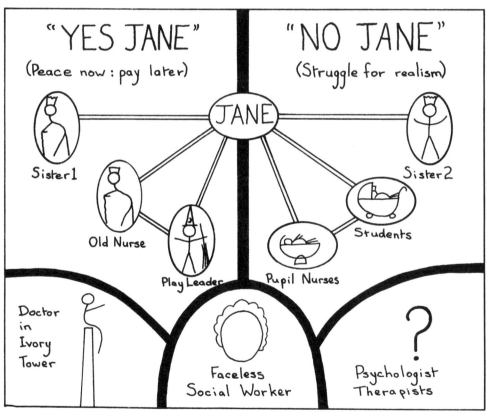

Management of Jane

difficult Jane and who were really firm with her (the students and pupils) were those who had little authority to act on her behalf. And as for the young Ward Sister 2, her good work was apparently undone by Sister 1 on the next shift. Both sides were managing Jane and thinking that they were doing it adequately, not realizing that one ('Yes Jane') was inadequate in the long-term, and doomed to make Jane more difficult. Neither saw that they were conflicting and therefore allowing Jane to manipulate them. The students and pupils at the bottom of the hierarchy, the ones who were with Jane most of the day, were only too aware of the effect the two conflicting approaches was having on Jane. Therapy staff, who might have evolved a programme of activities to help Jane, were well barricaded from the ward, in the students' drawing.

As they became more interested in what had seemed at first an exercise far removed from the examination syllabus, the students decided to delve into the question of whether the people who appeared to like Jane were in fact the people Jane approved of—an interesting investigation which no other group has considered. But having thought of it, the group found it too difficult to draw, and resorted to a simple diagram. Muddled as it was, it showed in startling fashion the confusion of Jane's world.

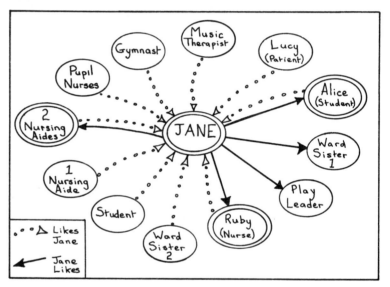

Who likes Jane—Whom does Jane like?

This was one of the rare groups who virtually refused to try cartoons, and the interesting problem of how it could be that the people who liked Jane were rarely those whom Jane liked, was never explored. It seemed that Jane liked those who gave in to her, the 'Yes Jane's.' Clearly, the students felt, Jane liked the 'bad managers' because she could manipulate them when she wanted her own way; and Alice (the student personally involved in the incident) shyly admitted here for the first time that she really *disliked* Jane, who made her feel incompetent.

Tutor and students found they were falling into the trap of discussing, rather than drawing, and in an attempt to break the circuit the question was introduced: Who had the knowledge, who the interest and who the power to help Jane?—She badly needed a training programme but was rejected by all the training units because of her behaviour. For once, the tutor drew the illustration, since the students still clung to the illusory security of words.

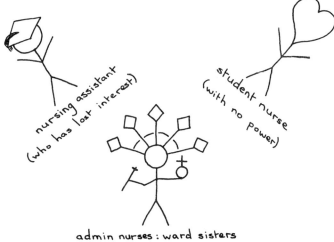

nursing assistant
(who has lost interest)

student nurse
(with no power)

admin nurses : ward sisters
(who have no knowledge)

Knowledge, power and desire to change

It was a new view of ward problems for the Cinderellas, and they were surprised to find that the three qualities were not present in any one member of staff. The next obvious question was: 'Why not?'

Relating it still to the ward situation and the incident, the group drew up a list of personal job satisfactions: what is it, they asked, that makes us say—'What a good day this has been!'? Perhaps this might help to explain the previous drawings.

We all know that job satisfaction is important. Without it, we become . . . bored? . . . frustrated? . . . grumblers? . . . aggressive? . . . apathetic? But what is job satisfaction, that lack of it gives us a headache at the end of the day instead of a pleasant glow of achievement? We need to identify, each one of us, *our own* personal goals so that we can then discover what it is that prevents us from achieving them.

The students, after a preliminary snort of: 'Money, of course—money and security!' settled down to produce a comprehensive list, meaningful to *them*, in *their* world (see page 62).

The students then ticked the personal satisfactions in working that had been present at the time of the incident for Alice, the student nurse concerned in the incident. Next, the group tried to imagine and assess the personal satisfactions of *other* members of the team: the ward sisters, the nurse administrator, the doctor, the social worker and the psychologist. It was a bold effort and one that required some encouragement. In doing it, the group started a new kind of exercise which subsequently produced some fascinating charts. The idea might well be expanded for assessing a total ward or departmental satisfaction (providing, of course, that it was done as an exercise arising from discussion of an incident and not starting from cold).

Alice's group imagined everybody's job satisfaction to be low, except the doctor's: his list was marked high on every aspect. He was seen as dedicated.

The nature of the work
variety
interest
crises dealt with calmly
day without stress
giving tender-loving-care
a sense of responsibility

Personal satisfaction
feeling wanted
having a sense of duty
someone depends on me
the day is too short
feeling efficient at something
security from deportation

Relationship with the client
dependency of patients
being of benefit to patients
getting thanks from patients
getting affection from patients
making patients happy
patients say: 'I'm glad to see you'
patients chatting to each other
patients prettily dressed
patients cheerful
not fearful

Relationship with other staff
getting praise from colleagues
getting thanks from seniors
working with pleasant colleagues
learning from one's colleagues

This is unusual since others have only been able to imagine that the doctor works for money—drawing him as the 'Rolls-Royce' consultant on page 74 or more simply, as a £ sign.

The whole class saw clearly now that *all* the staff on the ward received very little personal job satisfaction from Jane—and since there were several 'Janes' on this ward, morale was low. It took only a few moments for the young students to connect the low job satisfaction on this type of back ward with a number of problems such as poor communication between staff, and consequently poor service to the patients.

Now, too, the class could see for the first time that they were not the only ones to feel dissatisfied and frustrated: by imagining themselves into other people's shoes they discovered the high probability that most of the staff

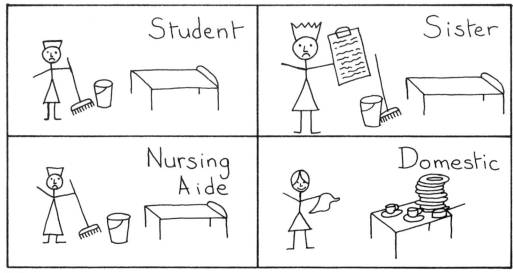

Roles

shared their feeling. Sympathy for the original 'villains' of the group became apparent.

A final attack was made on the iceberg, the hidden potential behind the original, simple incident.

The class, in drawing how each member of the ward team might see his role, found they had assigned that of domestic to everyone—the sister being distinguished only by doing a little paper work, while the domestic dallied with a little light dusting—*and*

Nobody was doing any *nursing*

The students then sat back and said: 'We want to do nursing!' A discussion followed on the topic: Why don't you have a ward run by students?

When the group discussed why there was such an emphasis on cleanliness, it was, of course, blamed on the nurse administrator. But when asked how things might develop if the students were allowed to run the ward as they wished, they said:

'But nothing would get done'
'Nothing of what?' asked the tutor
'No cleaning' replied the students
'Does it matter?'
'Yes' they answered
'To whom?' . . . (The students perhaps??)

The students were frightened that someone would have to carry the can, and that a weak person among them could jeopardize the careers of them all. It took them some time to discover that if they were all held collectively responsible, with appropriate leaders being thrown up at different times, then the team could function and support weak or recalcitrant members and see that priorities were upheld.

Finally the group discussed what mattered most in life, and what sort of things a parent would want to provide for his children. Loving and caring, giving attention and providing for material needs came much higher up the list than scrubbing and housework. Priorities were discovered not to be cleanliness after all.

During the four one-hour sessions these Cinderellas dealt with many complex and fundamental problems. They were able to see them illustrated in the ordinary, everyday world of their own wards. In this way, they began to recognize problems they had not been aware of. They also began to see constructive ways which they themselves could use to deal with these problems. These methods included rearousing the interest of the nursing assistant who (as seen on page 61) had the knowledge, by asking her advice about Jane; having the courage to speak up at ward meetings; and giving the weaker ward sister more practical support.

By the end of the course, the students no longer saw themselves as quite so impotent. They developed some understanding of the problems, role confusions and anxieties of other staff—both those more senior and those junior to themselves. No longer was the feeling so acute that what they learn in the training school is always unrelated or inapplicable to the ward setting.

The process of Illuminative Incident Analysis was probably most profoundly felt by Alice, whose incident this was, and she was able to admit to her own prejudices and frustrations. Painful conflicts which all the students had experienced (for instance, between play leaders and themselves) were seen with humour and with sympathy. Moreover, they recognized that some of the attitudes which they so heartily criticized in their seniors, were also raising their ugly heads in their own thinking.

Cinderellas maybe—but these students in a hospital for the mentally handicapped laboured with energy and persistence to produce this constructive analysis. We think there is enormous potential and energy among such Cinderellas which is often wasted in frustration while their contribution goes unrecognized. Perhaps other Cinderellas might also benefit (and so might the institution) if only they were seen as active participants in a team . . . and worthy of training in human skills.

Centre forward

In the Spider's Web diagram in chapter I we put the client, the patient, firmly in the centre of the team with an emphasis that might seem astonishing to those who have not themselves explored a number of incidents in this way. The idea was to remind ourselves and other professionals that there *was* a client.

In theory, the team is in existence solely to serve the client: in practice, the position often seems reversed. The hapless client serves as a focus for the team's problems, or is used as an outlet for their frustrations, or may virtually disappear from the scene as the unhappy team fights to work out its own destiny.

There are usually many threads in the tapestry, and we can only examine closely a few at a time. Various strategies appear in an unhappy team for using the client to conceal their own unhappy feelings. Here we consider two: 'tit-for-tat' and 'ignoring the patient.'

Tit-for-tat

Tit-for-tat has been present in many incidents already discussed, although, in order to keep the main theme clear we have not always drawn attention to it. From the Pink Daisies, bowling their incontinent subnormal women up and down the corridor between ward and unit, to the sad tale of Florrie, tit-for-tat has been there.

In the incident where Florrie was concerned, incredibly the warden of an old people's home ceased to communicate with the housing officer as a tit-for-tat gesture, paying her out because her favourite tablecloth had been used while she was away. Other aspects of Florrie tended to mask this, and, in that particular incident, were probably more important.

Unhappy staff, suffering from anxiety and unable to voice their feelings for one reason or another, bottle up their tensions for just so long until finally it becomes too much. They need an outlet. Unable to express themselves openly, or to halt the tide of new ideas and new faces in a changing organization, they may be diverted into manipulating their patients—quite without meaning any harm, and almost certainly unaware of what they are doing. In 'tit-for-tat' exercises staff are using the patient to express their own uncertainty. They are like two parents hurting each other through a third person—their child—and each manipulating the child to this end, without realizing that they are in fact quite unintentionally hurting the innocent victim (their child) in doing so.

Here we look in more depth at an obscure game of tit-for-tat which, had it been recognized at the time by senior staff, might have saved (as with the Pink Daisies) literally years of subterranean spite and management problems, exhausting in both time and emotions for a number of staff.

Sadie's Suppers
Incident: *Sadie lost her special privileges, through no fault of her own.* Sadie was a competent young woman in a long-stay hospital where she worked in a unit engaged in light industrial jobs. Here, Sadie was the best worker, responsible for checking the jobs before they were packed up for dispatch.

As a reward for her efficiency she was allowed by the supervisor to stay behind in the unit after the other patients had returned to the ward, and to join a select group for supper, chosen and cooked by themselves. This was a regular twice-weekly treat.

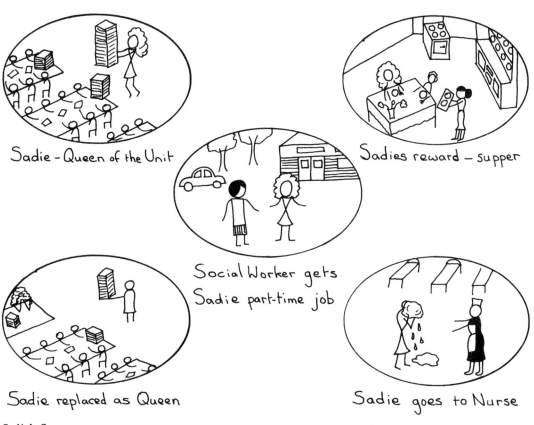

Sadie - Queen of the Unit

Sadies reward — supper

Social Worker gets Sadie part-time job

Sadie replaced as Queen

Sadie goes to Nurse

Sadie's Suppers

The time came when Sadie was found a part-time job outside the hospital by a new, young social worker. It was a pre-discharge exercise for this efficient and attractive patient. To minimize the possible strain of this new life, she continued working in the industrial unit in the hospital for the other three days.

But another, far less competent patient, was placed in charge of the checking counter. Sadie was put to work among the very inert, sick patients in another part of the unit. She was never again allowed to attend the special supper parties.

Sadie's upset took the form of withdrawal, and she spent her days on the ward, refusing to work in her new job or in the industrial unit.

On the surface, and to any inquirer, it might have seemed reasonable to find a new checker. So, too, could it be argued that the suppers were a privilege, a reward for good work. This is one of the subtleties of tit-for-tat: the affair often does seem reasonable until one remembers that a patient is suffering. In this case, at least three members of the team were aware of this: the supervisor in the industrial workshop; the social worker; and the ward sister.

The first drawings are an unusual feature of analysis in that the staff see the incident through the patient's (in this case Sadie's) eyes.

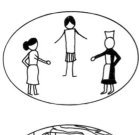

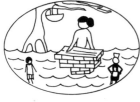

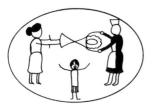

The picture was different when looked at from the staff angle. There was the bright, young, extroverted social worker, straight from college and full of new ideas for jobs in the community, leading to hostel care and finally, discharge. A kindly, protective, motherly ward sister now appeared in the drawings, whose patients were 'her babies'. Then there was the supervisor, whose unit had for twenty years been her private kingdom, before the unwelcome tide of new blood and new ideas began to lap at her doorstep. Her protective brick wall now crumbled away. Elderly, unqualified—and threatened by change, she seized the only retaliatory weapon her distorted emotions would provide: depriving Sadie of supper privileges. Ostensibly this was to hurt the social worker. In fact the only person who really got hurt was Sadie—whom the supervisor loved and protected. (She, too, called her patients 'her babies'.) Love's reverse is hate; and Sadie in the cradle became Sadie, the weapon to fight the world. Two women—and one 'baby' patient; and one young, attractive, qualified social worker with a husband and a baby, fighting for recognition in a hospital where progress had forced acceptance of a new style of staff. But the old staff did not desire the change, nor see the need for it. The infiltration of progress was imposed both from levels higher than the hospital and by public opinion; it could not be confronted, argued with or personalized. They did not know whom to fight or whom to hate, so they took it out on Sadie.

The incident severed the already delicate thread linking ward and unit staff. Sadie was removed from the unit by an indignant ward sister who assumed that Sadie's tears were caused by 'That Nasty Place Down There'. The social worker was, by that invisible decree so common in institutions, barred from that particular unit and was therefore unable to place any of those patients in outside employment for some time.

Similar in many ways to the Pink Daisies, Sadie's Suppers is a typical example of tit-for-tattery which, had it been worked on further, probably had equally deep roots in the original process of team-formation and in the 'high ideals-frustration-anger-apathy' sequence which is so worthy of further study.

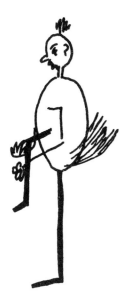

'You can't have **two** *things wrong!'*

Less intentionally malevolent, but nonetheless very serious for the patient is the strategy of ignoring, overriding, not listening to him. We see this most vividly when the incident concerns a second illness, or a second misfortune additional to the original problem.

Particularly in a shaky team, it is difficult enough to deal with one illness smoothly, let alone with two involving overlapping teams. Often it does not seem to enter anyone's head that two quite different hazards can occur simultaneously. This was the attitude when a wife brought her husband to the casualty department late one night and reported: 'He thinks he is a stork!'

There he stood, apparently brooding with knee clasped to chin. Silent, refusing to move his leg and so inaccessible to examination, he baffled the night staff, who could only take a blood sample and assume that his wife was right. He could see the psychiatrist in the morning. Too late, it was found that he was suffering, not from delusions, but from a ruptured stomach ulcer.

Another group of doctors was confronted with a docile little woman, admitted with a psychiatric illness to a general hospital, for drug therapy. Treatment commenced and seemed routinely satisfactory, but suddenly she went into a coma. It was the middle of the night. The young registrars on duty, summoned by the emergency call, clustered round muttering: 'She *can't* be really ill. She came in with phobic symptoms—and that's psychiatric!' But the docile patient was 'really ill,' and received a blood transfusion just in time to save her life.

A complaining, garrulous old lady in a geriatric unit was found after falling out of bed. Muttering: 'Wandering again—you naughty girl!' the nurse bundled her back to bed and tucked the blankets firmly in. 'Oh, my poor leg!' the old lady moaned all afternoon. But she was a regular complainer and no-body took any notice: she was, after all, senile. When a new night nurse came on duty, she looked at the leg and found it was four inches shorter than the other: the old lady had a fractured hip.

Another instance of ignoring the patient was entitled: 'Oh No, Not Him Again!'

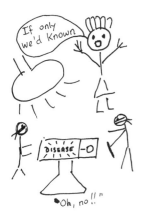

Originally Mr Jones was warmly welcomed to the ward with smiles and a cup of tea; introduced all round, he was made to feel at home. Admitted for just a minor operation, on recovering consciousness he continually asked for pain-killing drugs, crying that his stomach hurt. 'Always moaning,' the nurse cried eventually, as she smiled at the 'good' patient in the next bed, bearing up bravely without complaint. Busy with more serious cases, she by-passed his calls for drugs and was relieved when he was discharged home. A week later, he was readmitted. 'Oh no!' the ward sighed, 'not *him* again!' This time, carcinoma of the stomach was diagnosed. The nurse's remorse was almost unendurable.

None of these incidents, the various groups said, was due to understaffing, to lack of technology or skills. All concerned difficult, prickly patients, whom a busy team struggling to work together was only too glad to label with an easily identifiable diagnosis in order to simplify their handling of the person concerned. Why should the staff look for trouble? Difficult patients, like one's own difficult relatives or colleagues, make those around them anxious to avoid contact; it must be with a sigh of relief that suitable treatment for a recognizable illness can be initiated, leaving the hard-working staff free to pass rapidly on to a more rewarding patient or—since it can also happen in the social services—a client.

There can only be sympathy for staff trapped in this situation. In the end, with a troublesome, querulous, difficult patient, the priority becomes not the need to ameliorate his illness, but to keep him quiet. His physical, psychiatric or social needs assume less importance, and are ignored. Understandably.

Where is the patient?

There comes a time in the analysis of almost all incidents when the patient has disappeared from the drawings, or is at best a redundant figure around which the team are working out their own wrangles and misunderstandings. It happens in some drawings even, that the patient has been omitted completely—although by definition, the Illuminative Incident is one in which *the patient* has suffered some disservice. Often he is pushed to one side of the page, or is a tiny, obscure figure in relation to the rest of the team.

The Misfit

Incident: *a patient is sent down to the operating theatre, and the necessary equipment is not there.*

Mr Misfit was originally booked for Little Theatre A; the operation was changed for some reason to Big Theatre B. Nurse Jones, in charge of the ward, knew of the change, but when she went to coffee, Nurse Smith (who did not know) efficiently rang Little Theatre A to check that they were ready for Mr Misfit.

The Little Theatre A team were not ready. They panicked, and sent to Big Theatre B for the necessary equipment for the operation. Meanwhile, Nurse Jones returned from coffee, and immediately sent Mr Misfit down to Big Theatre B.

The equipment and Mr Misfit pass each other in the corridor, going in opposite directions. So when he arrives in Big Theatre B, the equipment is shining blissfully in Little Theatre A. Both theatre teams are exasperated, and time is wasted sorting out the muddle.

After several efforts at clarifying the incident, this is the group's final drawing of the complete team. In the Misfit, the patient is there, in the centre, cocooned and peacefully oblivious that the jigsaw of the team has somehow gone wrong. But he is not so vital that the picture would not fit together without him. Mr Misfit is recognized by the group as the centrepiece of the team, and they were making constructive efforts to move the two sides of the jigsaw together into one complete picture. It was a failed attempt, time as usual beating the constructive process. It was also a curious view of the patient as completely depersonalized.

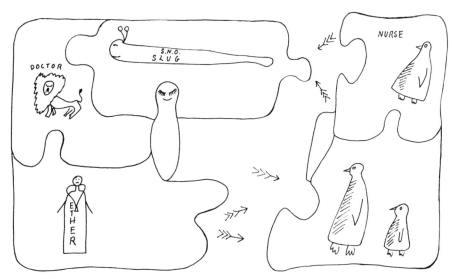

The Misfit

To summarize, we have concentrated in this chapter on some of the less palatable aspects of teamwork which the groups (whose incidents, after all, these are) have chosen themselves to examine. 'Dirt under the carpet,' this may be: we think it an important demonstration of wasted, under-used, mis-used human potential which could be developing many a vigorous and effective team.

One can only dimly imagine the frustrations and apathy of a highly-trained and intelligent person who is in a caring profession—and who has forgotten client and colleagues alike. For it is important to remember that these are neither fools nor malevolent people: they are members of a team of highly-skilled professionals, a team to which something has happened to destroy its harmony.

Where is your leader
Where is your team
and
Where is your client

?

6. Viewpoints

Objectives to the chapter

1. To take a close look, through their own drawings and cartoons, at the way nurses and doctors see themselves, each other and their patients—with a glimpse of engineer and pharmacist.

2. In this way, to understand some of the problems of role perception and attitudes that may hinder the healthy development of a team.

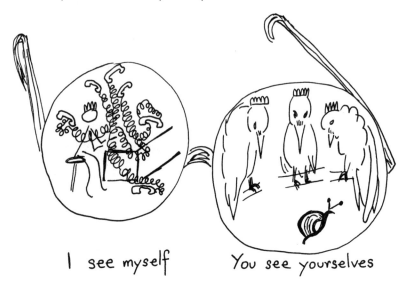

I see myself   You see yourselves

Just as the institution is more than a collection of buildings, so a team is more than a collection of people: both team and institution are fundamentally a conglomeration of human attitudes. Just as the highly qualified person who rises to the top of his profession is not necessarily a highly skilled leader, so the members of his team are not necessarily skilled in team work. Putting a group of people together, or listing them in a memo does not necessarily mean that we have a team which will automatically work as a team and stay as a team. Much will depend on their attitudes. In this chapter we examine how members of a team see each other—and their clients.

Whether I see you as a Devil with sharp horns and a spiky tail, or as a helpful, happy Angel, is going to colour my approach to you. Moreover, if you see yourself as a tiny Mouse, this will colour your response. Your reaction in turn, if you perceive me as 'God' will be quite different to your reaction if you see me as a Worm. It is a fairly safe bet, too, that you will not have considered how I am seeing myself; and only if I am unusually perceptive or honest, will I be aware of what I am—or of what you think I am. It makes a simple diagram.

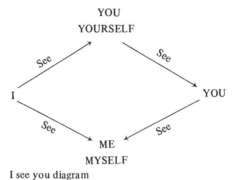

I see you diagram

This is the basis of role perception. It is an affair of expectations, emotions, previous experience and present events: reality takes second place. In considering roles, it is not what a person *is*, but how he is perceived by others that is important. And how people perceive is governed by their array of attitudes.

On the professional level, as contrasted with the personal level described above, it is only when you see me, for instance, as a psychologist whose job is to do intelligence tests, and I see myself in this same role, that our transaction will be smooth. For if you see this as my role, and I see myself as a psychologist who treats behaviour problems, leads group therapy, designs equipment or teaches staff, then we are *both* going to be frustrated. Because either I am going to be acting in a way which you are not expecting, and in a way which perhaps you don't want me to act; or I will conform to your expectations—and feel less job satisfaction. This is the straight, professional: I See You level. A relatively simple affair, it might be thought. We shall see a different view later in this chapter.

Firstly, we look at the more profound, elusive, emotional level—our attitudes. Taking various members of the team in turn, we start with the junior.

Group view

A-levels to L-plates

Why do they ever become student nurses? Why do they stay?

Juniors draw themselves with awesome inevitability surrounded by beds, baths, brooms, buckets and bedpans. Clothes-peg Peggy (in the Students'

World illustration) has just thrown away the last of a week's carefully hoarded samples of faeces: now the whole cycle will have to be repeated, and the wretched patient is doomed to spend another week on the bedpan. Slops and sluices: menial jobs maybe, but the hapless student is often galloping through a minefield. For the menial job may require knowledge which the student has not yet acquired, in order to avoid disaster: in this case the student was not aware that a week's total faeces is required for a faecal fat count.

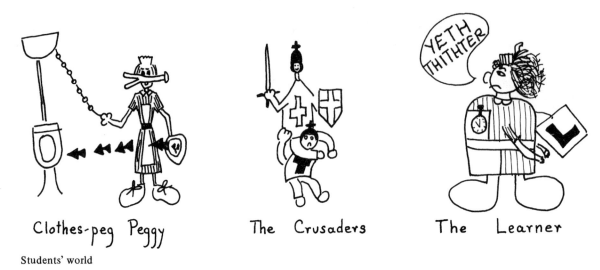

Clothes-peg Peggy   The Crusaders   The Learner

Students' world

When a student answers a telephone inquiry from Mrs A. Bloggs, she doesn't yet realize that she should call her senior to the telephone (or maybe she was too scared to interrupt the ward round)—and in proud ignorance she reports that Mr Bloggs has just died. How was she to know there were two Mr Bloggs— and that Mr A. Bloggs was tucked up happily in bed, while Mr B. Bloggs had just died? How was she to know that *this* Mrs Bloggs would take the hospital to court and receive a sum in compensation for the shock and distress she was caused?

In the long-stay hospital, students drawing themselves as crusaders feel that they are the only members of the team who are actively on the patients' side, battling for the patients' rights. And even as crusaders they are forced to support one another, student riding upon the back of student. Senior staff, they think, have other priorities: they are the ward managers, no longer caring staff.

Students are in a state of perpetual conflict; learning a highly respected profession with new and exciting techniques, requiring a high educational standard—while performing the daily routine of menial and unpleasant jobs. The paradox lies in the fact that, despite their subservient position, they feel themselves to be closer to the patient (because of these bed-and-bathing tasks) than those who are managing the wards and supervising treatment. And in some ways, they *are* in a better position to be the patient's friend, to be confided in, to notice subtle differences in condition. *But* they are without the skills and experience to sift out what is important.

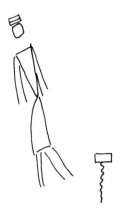

Often, a student comes straight from the sixth form and has passed a number of exams to get into the training school. This is her big moment. Freed from the schoolgirl image, she is now *a nurse*. Yet she finds another kindergarten. From being a big fish in a little pool, she is once again among the tiddlers of the nursing pond, complete with L-plate.

'Clean their teeth!' says sister, finding junior unoccupied during the night hours. A moment's anxiety ('Am I doing it right? Better not ask!') and junior tips the ward's teeth into one large bowl; and soon rows of shining teeth are laid neatly upon the table for sister's inspection. Unfortunate junior! For sister is faced next day with the humiliating task of asking relatives: 'Are *these* your mother's teeth?' And twenty sets of unidentifiable teeth finally have to be replaced at the hospital's expense.

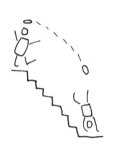

Unsure by now of what she does know, the ex-sixth former ponders. Ought she to know? Has she forgotten? Did she fall asleep in class? Did she get her notes down correctly? . . . Junior now sees her senior as an awesome figure in the hierarchy. Frightened to reveal her ignorance, she also fears her senior's anger. And, for the junior, the senior is seen as an unappeasable, unapproachable, sizable figure of starch. A Lady Chieftain.

It is an apprenticeship of tears which few of her contemporaries are prepared to accept.

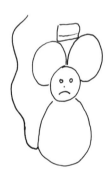

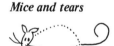

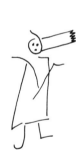

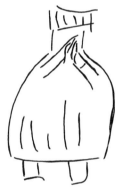

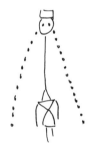

Mice and tears

In stark contrast, the senior sees a different picture. 'She ought to know!' she thinks to herself, 'She spends enough time in that school!' And, as the cartoon of nurse in a 'tizzy' showed us, sister may genuinely be too busy, too short of staff in a crisis, to think to tell her junior such apparently simple details as: 'Remember to clean each set of teeth separately!'

What the junior does not realize is the latent sympathy of her seniors. Perhaps it is not normally at the forefront of their minds, but in the emotional context of analysing an incident, sister, tutor and administrator can all produce highly sensitive drawings—and often see with a sense of shock just what is happening to their junior staff.

What we need to find out, is how to keep these drawings at the forefront of the senior's mind, to signpost her daily attitude to her students. Sister, at least, sees herself in her role as a senior as wholly responsible for her juniors—whatever the consequences of the junior's actions. Sister has to face the music. Sister has her own apprehensions and fears, as we see in the next chapter when we ask: Who supports the nurse?

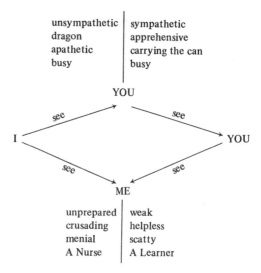

Four-way perception

Junior and senior: each in turn is misperceiving the other, attitudes coloured by emotions. Will the juniors in their turn treat their students in the same way, with similar misperceptions? 'I hope I don't', one junior said, 'but I'm very much afraid I shall be like all the other seniors. I shan't be able to help it!' Because the same pressures will come to bear on her as did on her seniors she will give way like they did—unless she has had the foresight to build her own supportive team.

Doctors

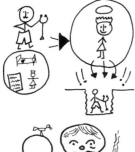

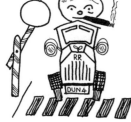

In the drawings, barbed wire often separates the doctor from the rest of the team; equally, he may be isolated on Cloud 9. Cartooned as an ostrich with head in the sand, marooned on one side of the paper as in the Four Sons, the doctor is a lonely figure, even if seen as lonely by choice. Seldom is the doctor seen as a closely supported—or supporting—member of the team. In this illustration of a junior doctor, he sees himself as efficient and above the ward, literally in charge and certainly superior. In the ward's eyes, however, he is 'firmly squashed' by sister and reduced to size. Sweet revenge! Consultants are even further removed in the hierarchy. 'Rolls-Royce' was done by an engineer working on an incident with a senior management group and interpreting their comments on the opulent consultant. If this is the attitude towards the medical member of the team, how can there be a warm and effective working relationship? No wonder this incident split a team down the middle.

A lot has been said earlier about the tradition of the doctor as leader of a team: the doctor, as he appears in most drawings, still has to learn the skills of working as a member of a team. Doctors seldom, as yet, join in exercises such as these; from those who have done so we show two drawings which suggest how some see their nurses.

The brick wall may seem an unsympathetic image to use to depict a member of a caring profession, but at least the group of doctors producing this drawing is sensitive to the nurse's feeling of being subservient to the medical profession. And, with some humour, sensitive to the reason why she takes it out

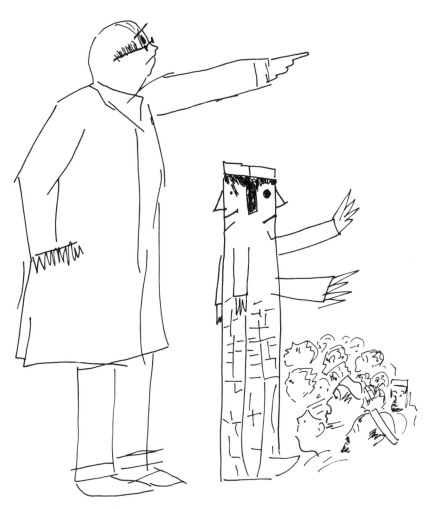

Doctor—nurse—patient

on the patients. This is another version of the Two-headed Nurse: subservient to the dominating medical figure—and dominating in turn—the masses, the patients at floor-level. Equally sensitive is the image of the Clockwork Nurse, for although he does not see her as a real person but as an uninvolved object, at least he is aware of not involving her—and once again, in vivid and unforgettable imagery.

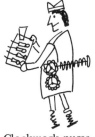

Clockwork nurse

If the doctor's attitude towards his nursing team is to see them as automatons, not humans, he is building his expectations of cooperation on a picture that cannot possibly be maintained. He is expecting his nurses to give the efficient service of a machine; nurses (it should not need to be said) are *human*.

How can you talk to a hedgehog?

The richest variety of caricatures comes when a group of staff of any kind draws the patient.

In moments of stress, patients obviously provoke a great variety of emotion. If any one of the following drawings expresses your attitude towards someone in your care, there will be problems in giving him support, whatever your profession—and if we are honest, we have all experienced this kind of attitude towards our clients, whoever they may be.

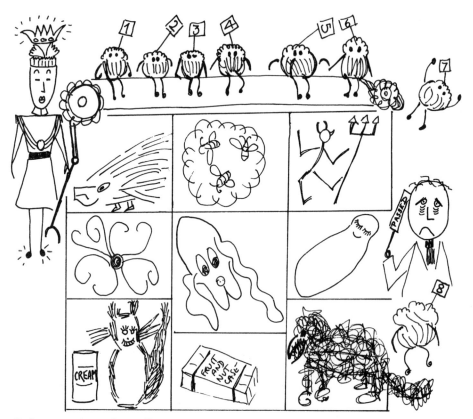

Patients—as drawn by staff

Shocked perhaps, or like the nurse in the Four Sons, energetically and understandably concealing from yourself these unacceptable feelings, how much time can you spare for consideration of the other side of the picture: how your patient sees you? Little enough in all probability, since staff of any kind rarely draw themselves as they imagine their patients see them.

It is, of course, unreal to see your patient as a hedgehog: but if this is how you *feel* about her, it is going to colour your attitude towards her and your communication with her—look at the lines of non-communication with Tracy, in the Queen Bee. You might even go out of your way to avoid her, because

76

her spines are sharp and painful—and anyway, how do you talk to a hedge-hog? Even so, to admit that:

'I see you as a prickly hedgehog!' is one thing.
'How does this hedgehog see me?' is a more difficult concept.
And the logical question: 'Am I somebody's hedgehog?' is an unbearably painful one.

It is scarcely more dignified to approach your patient as if he were a basset hound. This, too, is likely to present problems of attitude and communication, since you are regarding him as something of a pet—and perhaps, like the group who drew this illustration, you, also, will think of yourself as a dispenser of juicy marrow bones for good behaviour. More subtle a danger, but a dangerous attitude nonetheless.

The terror of technology

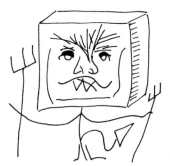

Advances in medicine and advances in machinery: what does it do to a caring team if 'I See You' as a machine? In this particular instance, drugs were ordered through some kind of computer system not fully understood by a junior. Fortunately, the incident only involved a duplicated order. The cartoon, however, highlights the removal of an already remote part of the team—the dispensary—to the realms of unreality. Communication with huts and units, laboratories and workshops sited at a distance from the wards, is difficult enough: communication with a machine is an affair of drab efficiency almost bound to result, sooner or later, in bitter ill-feeling and wasted energy.

Chorus: 'We see ourselves . . .'

If you are a nurse in charge of a busy ward, the chances are you see yourself like this. No time for planning, for attending to your patients individually—or their relatives, no time for training your juniors. But for all of us, whatever our job in the health or social services, *this* is the epitome of our martyred view

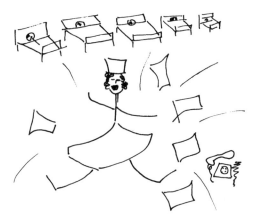

of our own working lives. And if all our energy has to be concentrated on bearing up under the burden of duty, how can we have anything to spare for consideration of the rest of the team? We are not going to be of much service to our fellow team members if we see ourselves thus:

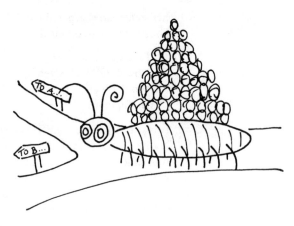

But how do the others see us? Such drawings as the next are not uncommon. They pose a problem. If even simple attitudes about how much work one does, or how idle one is, are so improbable—with what clarity of purpose can we hope to work together?

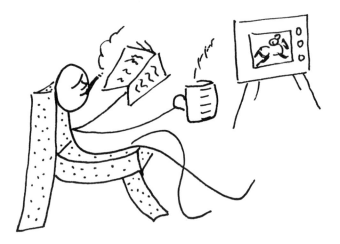

Which way do we look?

Whatever the complications of attitudes, there is another ingredient of communication to be considered: roles. Though perhaps not so emotionally coloured as attitudes, roles are not static and in some professions seem to be particularly hard to pin down. What is, for instance, the role of the nurse? Is she a scientific observer of symptoms and changes, a comforter, a dispenser of drugs? Is she a teacher? Is she a manager or a machine? And even if I, as her colleague, do realize that she has several roles, how do I discern which role she is in at this particular moment? We have seen the dilemma of the two-headed nurse: should she rush to cope with a patient or, as a manager, delegate? It is often more complex than this.

For example, the nurse in a hospital for the mentally handicapped may see her role as that of educator, in the broadest sense as a parent educates his child. But if her colleagues in the team do not realize that she sees this as her role two consequences will confuse communication. Firstly, those who could advise and help her in her role of educator, will not see the necessity to do so: the teacher may have books and educational toys that would be useful, but he does not think of lending them. The psychologist could offer experience of learning theory—but hesitates to do so. There may be voluntary workers available for help with mastering money, reading or time . . . but they will not be asked to visit the ward. All this can easily happen because others do not think of the nurse in the role of educator. But secondly, her colleagues *are* seeing her in some role or other—and often each in a different one. Each, then, will have different expectations and therefore make different demands upon her. And often all at the same time.

Poor nurse! Playing Pygmalion and seen as Florence Nightingale; or even worse, longing to be Florence Nightingale and forced to play *Dad's Army*. No job description, no list of nursing duties can really signal to *us*, her colleagues, which role at which moment any one of the nurses on ten, twenty, thirty—or even forty wards in the hospital, is playing.

There is another side to the picture: our colleagues, seeing us—or even needing us—in one particular role, may confine us to that role almost against our will. A role, maybe, which we have long outgrown as techniques have advanced. We all experience to some extent these conflicting expectations and realities. But, once again, it is the nurse who experiences the extremes, and the greatest multiplicity of viewpoints.

One man's telescope

A solo attempt to clarify roles and interpersonal relationships on his ward was made by Ben, a young student nurse in his second year. His growing awareness illustrates constructively the use of an Illuminative Incident as a self-teaching instrument by a junior. Ben thought the incident a trivial one, he was unsure of its value and apologetic. Yet it had angered him.

Cakes for Tea

Incident: *Students' attempts to give residents on a ward cakes for tea, instead of for supper, were thwarted.*
Two eager student nurses in a hospital for the mentally handicapped, came to the ward fresh from lectures on 'normalization'. Treat the patients as you would treat any normal human being, they were told; patients have a right to dignity—and they will rise to your expectations.

The students looked at the patients' menu in the ward kitchen: cakes for supper. 'Let's make cheese sandwiches for supper', they said, 'and have the cakes for tea, just like we do at home.' They laid the cakes daintily on the tea-table.

The staff nurse came along. 'Cakes on the menu for *supper*, it says—and cakes for supper it is!' And the students had to clear the cakes away.

Trivial maybe. But Ben nearly left his job: it was the last straw in the daily conflict between what he was taught in the training school and the monotonous reality of the wards.

The first analysis was in writing, and sound though it was, Ben felt he had learned nothing from it; he had known it all before he started.

1. Student nurses want to start new things, often just for the sake of doing something new (progress, in their eyes) and usually to the annoyance of the charge nurse ('I've a good routine, a stable ward.') Consequently, students tend to do things under cover, without informing anybody.

2. Charge nurse may have thought that new suggestions were a criticism of his ward, which he had brought up from a low standard and fought hard to maintain.

3. Staff nurse—young and newly qualified, was eager to follow the correct procedure. Popular with everyone, a likable person, and greatly admired by the charge nurse.

4. Kitchen boy—an adult patient who was now totally in charge of the ward kitchen. He did not like staff to interfere with his work, even if it meant that patients had sub-standard meals (e.g., cold tea)—though admittedly this did not happen often.

The second stage took the form of drawing, in an attempt to get away from the bondage of words. Ben chose to illustrate separately the points of view of each of the four main characters in the incident. He did this in a dramatic and simple way. It was Ben's own idea, and it was the first time that such a complex exercise in empathy had been tried.

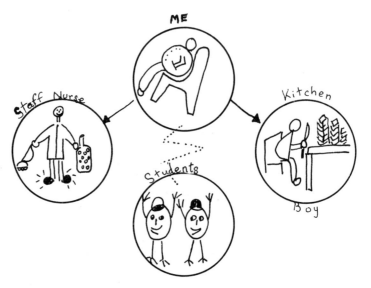

i. *Charge nurse*

'I can sit back now. My ward is organized. The staff nurse is in control and Tommy is making tea . . . But what are those two little beasts up to?'

The third stage was a detailed look at the charge nurse. Ben had used the phrase 'running on oiled wheels' when speaking of the ward, and he sketched a cartoon-style illustration of what the charge nurse wanted his ward to be. Tweedledum and Tweedledee (the two students) were now drawn as puppies, firmly on a lead. This brought home vividly to the authors the skill needed

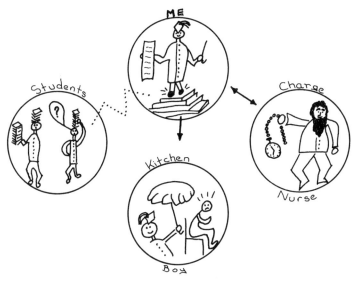

ii. *Staff nurse*

'Well I'm fully qualified now and must show those poor students what to do. I must take the burden off the charge nurse—but keep to his timetable and protect poor Tommy in the kitchen.'

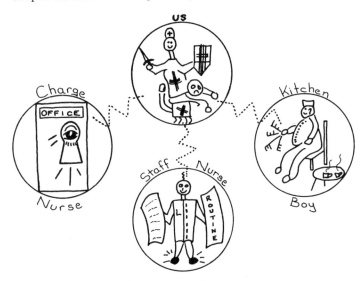

iii. *Two student nurses*

'We're Crusaders, going to change things for progress. But we'll have to watch out in case *he* sees us. How are we going to get to the cakes when Tommy is guarding them? The staff nurse won't help, he's looking for a charge nurse post and keeping his shoes clean.'

by the nurse in charge of a ward to balance his staff and patients and students in this way—and it highlighted the problem of conflict between managerial and patient-centred skills. It also demonstrated clearly his fears and anxieties as the changes of the new Health Services Act in 1974 approached and threatened (he thought) to upset his balance on his bicycle.

We then discussed this blanket-term 'change'. Ben told us that in many wards the psychologists, for instance, were seen as outsiders bent on causing trouble. Linked as we were with new ideas on education and training of the patients,

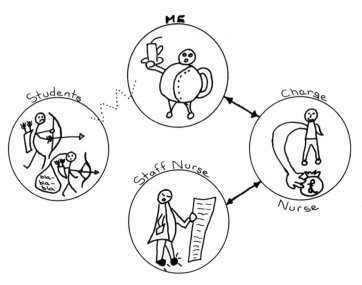

iv. *Kitchen boy*

'I'm a good kitchen boy. I make the charge nurse cups of tea, he gives me money. I don't like those students upsetting my job, I don't understand what they say. Anyway, staff nurse agrees with me.'

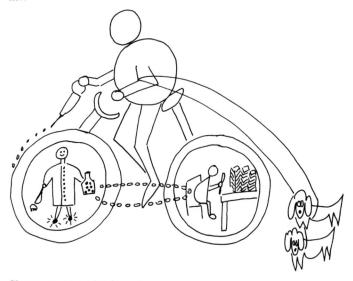

Charge nurse on his bicycle

82

we thought this could, just possibly, be how we were seen—but it wasn't true, we said, indignantly.

Ben's next illustration shattered us.

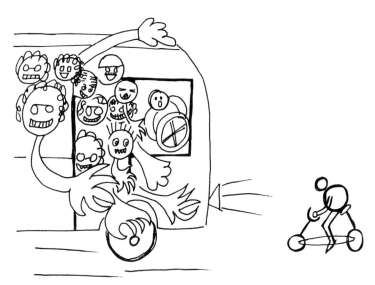

Crash course

He saw us as part of a sizable group of staff, all fairly recently appointed, all with new ideas and fresh enthusiasms. Democratically led by a consultant psychiatrist, at times it could be asked: 'Who *is* your leader?'

It was a drawing of ourselves as others saw us which, from sheer shock, resulted in action.

Together, Ben and the authors tried to find ways of preventing the collision and Ben chose to use the illustration of a railway station (firmly rejecting our idea of a troika driven by the nurse, with three equal horses: students, nurse administration and innovator-therapists). The exercise was a difficult one for all of us.

> 'Who is going to be the guard?'
> 'We've left the doctor out!'
> 'Make him station announcer?'
> 'That's not a very important role.'
> 'The signalman—now *he* has an overall view. Who should he be? Not the doctor . . . but who does have an overall view?'
> 'The psychologists (said Ben) seem to know where the train *might* be going, and where the junctions are. So should they be the signalman, or the guard—or the timetable, or . . . what?'

Telescopic viewpoint
Ben says this has been an exercise in empathy. He has learned not to take the surface view, but to respect other, different attitudes. Suddenly, he has realized how confined and cut-off his world is on the ward, peopled only by nurses, ward orderlies and domestics. Our world, teeming with therapists,

social workers, training staff, teachers, doctors and administrators in on a different planet.

In future, he thinks he will see the ward as he has drawn it, with the various viewpoints, and will look for the underlying structure with some understanding. Though Ben is doubtful whether he could use the technique as a staff nurse, he certainly will when he has his own ward to run.

The authors, psychologists in Ben's hospital, learned a lot from watching his struggles to clarify his own incident. For the first time they have a sharp realization of the world of the charge nurse, balanced so delicately and efficiently on his bicycle. His skill is vividly depicted in Ben's drawing. And now they fully realize just what they, and the other innovators, are doing to him. Far from being 'members of a team' they are unleashing the 'eager puppies' (believing as they do that the students are the strength of the institution) and causing a head-on collision. The coach is loaded with grimly determined people: something has to be done, with some urgency, to save coach and bicycle from a crash which could prove fatal to both.

It is interesting to contemplate the unmistakable conclusion that none of us—and between us we represented top management, middle management and the learners—had any real idea of roles. Who could be the planner, to prevent the crash; who the leader; who the driver? Who represents the energy in the team, and who the power?

One might suppose it to be essential for any learner to be given a clear map of the institution he is to work for and study in. It would without any doubt astonish those at the top to find the learners floundering in this way. Ben, in his second year, is a mature, active and involved student yet, like other students before him, he is clearly astonished by the size of the team *outside* the ward.

We, the psychologists, were equally astonished to discover that the team we belong to is so wrapped in fog as to be virtually non-existent in the eyes of the ward—the centre of the patients' world.

While it could be argued that this feeling of being cocooned in the ward is a factor of the student's inexperience, professionally these are the impressionable and formative years. If students like Ben believe, as he shows in this exercise, that the ward team consists for all practical and visible purposes of nurses and domestics (and patients), this will set the pattern for the whole of his future thinking, as it has done for generations past. As a result students can only develop a clannish outlook that will be difficult to eradicate. Who will open the students' eyes? How will Ben and other students like him, in turn influence their students?

We, on the other hand, believed, before this exercise, that we worked in a highly involved, multi-disciplinary setting that was widely publicized through meetings, newsletters and discussions.

It may be that the whole learning programme should be turned upside down and the first-year student be attached to each *member* of a multi-disciplinary team in turn, for several weeks. And only then be allocated to a ward or a department. Might it not be more effective for our clients if we deliberately developed team-thinking *before* professional skills and not afterwards, when the isolation of one discipline from another is already an entrenched attitude?

Ben's work on this minor incident demonstrates impressively his discoveries of the hidden structure of the institution, and its strengths and weaknesses. We ourselves have never, in formal lectures or even in discussions, been able to bring out such rich insight. Without the technique of drawings and cartoons we have found apathy and resignation creeping in. Ben, and other students who have become involved in Illuminative Incident Analysis, are less inclined to say: 'You can't'. Their attitude becomes one of constructive questioning: 'How can we succeed, what do we need to do, who can help?'

We don't know why this is. Ben himself said he would never have acquired such insight had he not analysed in this way his own, personal incident in such depth. What we cannot explain is why being prevented from giving out cakes for tea should trigger off such a valuable learning process.

'I'm really concerned', Ben said later, 'I must find out what lies behind these attitudes. Because it is the constant, daily repetition of these incidents that begins to frustrate and depress.'

Panorama

Occasionally a group will analyse their incident in breadth and encompass many diagnostic and remedial points in one illustration. The Four Sons and Wobbly Jelly seem to have a universal appeal and make excellent demonstration material. The Sausage is another such incident and its rough drawing makes the unmistakable point that you don't have to be an artist to express your feelings (see page 86).

The Sausage

Incident: *a patient choked on a sausage and died.*
Mrs Jones was diabetic and in a comatose state when lunch came round. It was sausage and mash, and the student nurse—only just out of her introductory lectures in the training school—wondered whether it was all right to give it to her. She had never before seen anyone comatose. She went back to ask sister.

Sister, coping with a busy surgical ward at lunch time, was accustomed to having senior students and didn't realize just how inexperienced this new junior was. Brusquely, she told her to go ahead.

Frightened, but assuming that Mrs Jones was just rather miserable, the young nurse left the plate of food on the bed tray. Mrs Jones, dazed, tried to feed herself, choked on the sausage and died.

The presenter of the incident was the sister concerned, and it is intriguing to notice the different styles of drawing her. Without needing any depths of interpretation, it is clear that she becomes more and more primitive in the drawing, losing first her uniform, then her face and arms, and is finally reduced to just a line. Junior, too, is seen as a fairly big person who rapidly shrivels on being given her first Real Job. And which of us has not felt like the third picture!

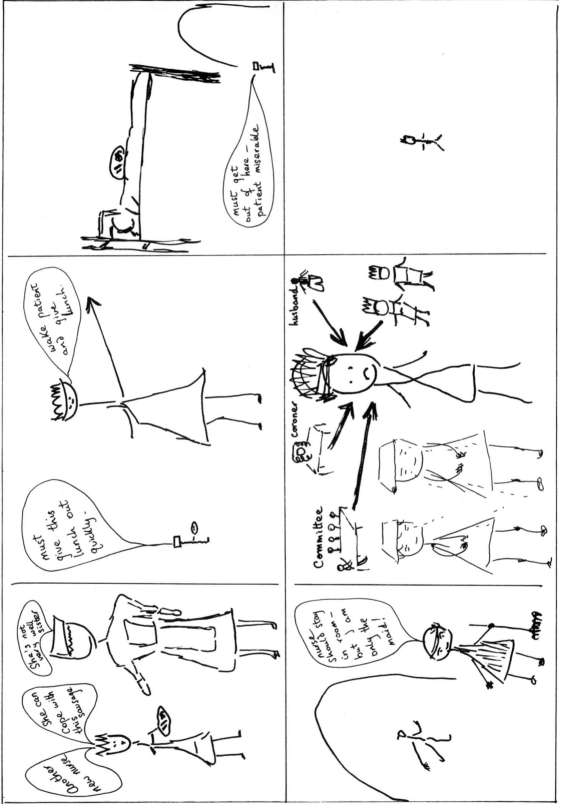

The Sausage

A point which crops up over and over, is The Little Man Who Knows (but doesn't say). The porter, the receptionist, the telephonist, the ambulance driver . . . all in fact vital supporters of the team because they *are* the people who hear rumours, who pick up odd bits of knowledge, who see patients, relatives, staff, neighbours—and perhaps, too, they are people with time to listen. In the Sausage, it is the domestic who is The Little Man. Experienced if not qualified, she knows enough to know when something is wrong. But: 'it's not *my* job to speak!' An apathy, a resentment perhaps, that is born of long years of seeing herself (if not being seen) as the nobody at the bottom of the hierarchical ladder—if, in fact, she even reaches the ladder at all. And certainly the student does not see her as a source of knowledge, advice or comfort.

Another familiar thread binding the patchwork of incidents: sister always gets the blame. Or sees herself this way. Illustrations of sister surrounded by a fence of accusing fingers, by judge, coroner, management committee, seniors and relatives, appear with the regularity of nightmares before exams. In the Sausage, the guilt is there as well: two pathetic orphans. This is sister's world as she sees it.

It is this final Sausage picture which should be pinned over the desk of every member of every hospital team—and given to every patient and every relative. In its stark loneliness it is the most haunting of all our drawings. Who supports the ward sister in her moment of trouble? Who is there to advise her, to pick up the pieces, to allay her anxiety, to help her to live with her feelings of guilt? Sister herself sees nobody.

Perceptions of ourselves and others, of attitudes and roles, are not static affairs of fact. If we in the team can be constantly alert to changes and developments in 'How I See You' in all its facets, then our contacts with each other will be more productive. Our energy will not then be dispersed on the chimera of false imaginings and needless blame.

Are *you* somebody's hedgehog?
Does someone need your support?
Can you do a 'Cakes for Tea?'

Part 3—Action learning

7. Exploration

Objective to the chapter

To present aspects arising out of analysing
Illuminative Incidents by drawing—aspects which
seem to us to raise questions for deeper study in
the future.

To reduce the original incident to cartoon form complete with useful insight
into the team and its members, and with perhaps a few constructive suggestions
for action, is a goal which can be attained in one or two sessions. However, a
wealth of enticing detail may have been passed over, all of which will certainly
reveal more problems, as well as further avenues for exploration of the team's
fundamental structure.

There are an infinite number of possible variations, but we offer the following as a starting point, since we feel they are key issues, particularly in large
institutions. There are questions which have a certain urgency, such as: Who
supports the nurse? Who is in the patient's world? There are practical guide-
lines which indicate the earliest possible moment for action: *a vade mecum*
which we have called 'danger signals'.

The careless comment: 'Well, sister should have known anyway', and the
rough drawing of a tiny termite of a student nurse scuttling from the room;
the parents who are spoken of, yet never appear in the drawing, and the
grave dug by sister who towers over a shrivelled junior doctor drawn huddled
in the trench—all are indications of a hidden depth to the story.

Who supports the nurse?

Some of the drawings done by our groups are neat and factual, some pure
scribble; some are static, some have movement; some are crowded and some
empty. Some, like the series in the Sausage, start in one style and become
increasingly primitive as the drama develops. Whether nurse is trim and
efficient, drawn with the precision of the professional illustrator, or is a
hopeless, bewildered tangle of wobbly, tentative lines, in one way or another

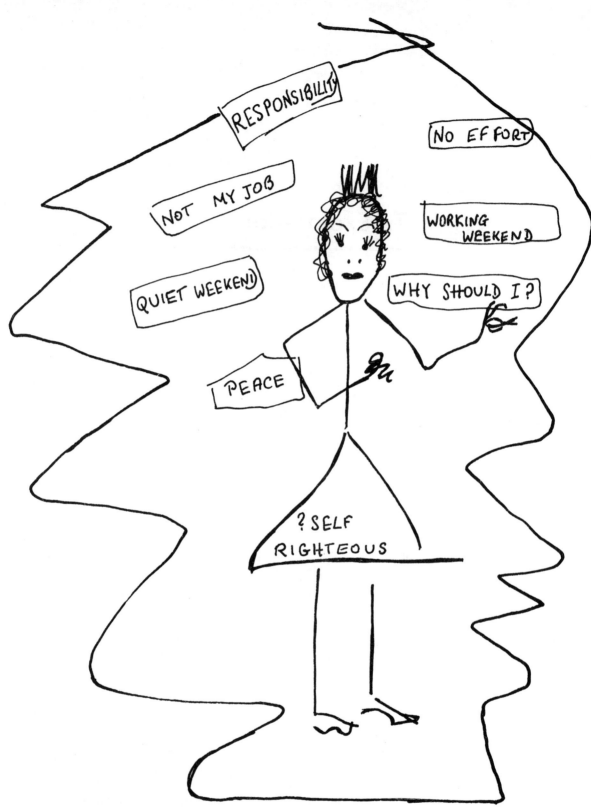

Danger signals from unsupported nurse

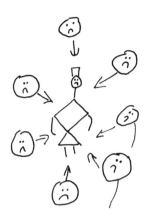

the group frequently make one thing clear: in a moment of crisis the nurse sees herself alone, unsupported.

The frightened student in the Sausage, crawling through a hole in the wall, and the lonely ward sister feeling herself abandoned after the inquiry, both embody the theme. The comfortable, experienced nurse in the Four Sons stands, a tiny speck in one corner, with the three consultants together at the furthest opposite corner of the paper. In this drawing the hospital management committee is busy fencing the nurse in with accusing fingers: who is on her side?

In the next drawing, again she is alone—with the committee clustered together in comfortable plurality. This nurse is taking the blame for a doctor's omission: 'You have to cover up', she says. But she is bitter—and alone. to an understanding of what has gone wrong.

The third drawing seemed commonplace enough: the overburdened nurse. But this nurse, in illustrating it literally, had a flash of insight: 'No wonder,' she she said, 'that I feel so tired always.' Or again, the Centipede Nurse, bearing bedpan and bottle, scurrying in a hundred directions simultaneously.

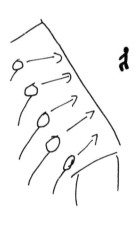

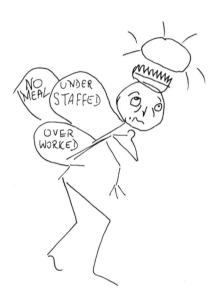

Overburdened nurse

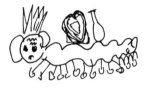

The nurse's paradox: emotion boiling up and over, outwards towards colleagues and patients; and emotion welling up within, turning to helpless tears. It's the old nurse story: angel or devil; giant or mouse; tears or anger; efficiency or helplessness.

Few professions can produce such contradictory states: the demand for miracles, the need for perfection—and the reality of human ignorance and error; birth and death; routine and emergency; caring but impassive.

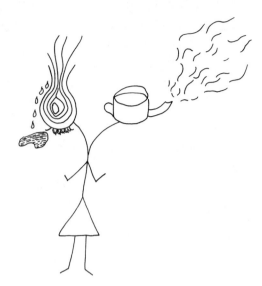

The kettle and the onion

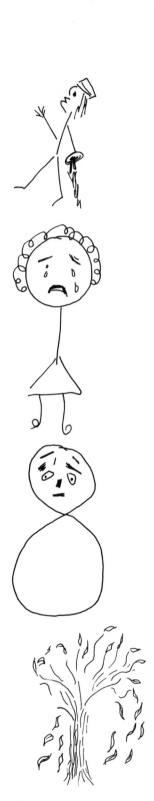

It starts with hard work and the disenchantment of bedpans and bottles, and soon we have the Frightened Nurse. Nothing very serious at this stage. But it comes, almost inevitably, to what is shown in the drawing. It doesn't really need an art therapist to tell you that this is an expression of grief. And whether you would agree or not, both art therapist and psychologist would suggest that you consider the absence of arms—in a nurse whose very profession of caring demands that she reaches out to help. This time, nurse cannot even reach out *for* help, for herself.

How much deeper, then, is the next expression of how a nurse sees herself. This one is drawing her feelings after a patient died. Its sensitivity of helpless, wild grief, despite (or because of) the childish drawing, is clear. This is grief and depression, frozen and immobile. Not even a tear this time, nor arms, nor legs. Who *does* support her? And finally, the Withered Tree bears repetition: the ultimate in despair. But this time, the senior, too, shared in the emotion of the young student who sent the wrong Mrs Jones to the operating theatre: *her* students will receive counselling in future.

Nurse counselling is still a new conception and money for research even on an 'action learning', do-it-yourself scale is hard to come by. Many nurses don't ask for it, for various reasons. Many senior staff—nursing or medical—don't offer it. It is no easy task, and, perhaps understandably, the most perceptive among us are not always in the mood to take on other people's troubles.

We have met so far over a thousand people in the setting of Illuminative Incident Analysis and have several hundred drawings. We think the question:

Who supports the nurse?

to be the most urgent among those we have unearthed for further exploration.

94

Tommy's world

A technique of exploration which we sketched out in chapter 1, the Spider's Web team, put the client or the patient firmly at the centre, and linked those dealing with him to each other, to give mutual support in the often emotionally demanding work of a caring profession. This technique is developed here.

An incident, when it arises, belongs to that particular moment in time, and involves probably only a limited number of people from the team serving that particular patient. There are, of course, many others who may be deeply concerned and who are vital to an understanding of what has gone wrong. They may also have quite different views of his needs. One way of exploring behind the presenting problem, of breaking out of the rigid here-and-now structure and using a creative approach, is to consider who is in that particular patient's world. We personalize him here as 'Tommy'.

Tommy is the most important member of the team. We sometimes forget that without him not only would there be no incident, but no team—and no jobs for us, the professionals. Tommy's interaction with team members is of vital importance. Putting Tommy in the centre with the team revolving round him is one way of looking at it, but making him an important and active member of the team—particularly in long-stay hospitals—is another. This avoids the familiar complaint of Tommy himself, that activity is going on all round him but that he, the patient, the vital person, is not part of it.

People outside the immediate situation in hospital, hostel or home, may be extremely important to Tommy in his world, if not to the professionals in theirs. His employer, for instance, his colleagues, neighbours, the landlord of his local may be key figures and case conferences have often been enriched by their presence.

The first time this was done, in a long-stay hospital, a class of student nurses had been stirred from their 'you are here to *teach* us!' mood sufficiently to grumble in the usual fashion about lack of staff, lack of money, overcrowding—and the inevitable whipping boy—the laundry. Urged to be more positive, the students went blank and reverted to 'They'. Meetings between ward and laundry were suggested by the tutor, and the idea met with a shuffling of feet and a 'Yes, but . . .'

So the tutor started doodling with a spider's web, placing the therapeutic team close to Tommy and the administrators on the fringe. Suddenly and spontaneously a lively exchange of ideas developed:

> 'You've left out Tommy's friends!'
> 'Yes—they're right there in the centre, they should be. *They're* the people who stand up for him.'
> 'It's his friends who give him *companionship*, not us.'
> 'He *learns* from his friends.'
> 'His friends *understand* him—even if he can't speak.'

Tommy's friends, the class insisted, are part of the therapeutic team, at least, in a long-stay hospital. And when Tommy is transferred from one ward to another, or (more important) from one hospital to another, his friends should go with him.

An interesting session evolved on teaching and training the mentally handicapped, and on policy for hostels and discharge. As so often happens, drawing and doodling released some hidden energy that was otherwise being dispersed in negative grumbles.

In exploring Tommy's world, we can return to those important questions raised briefly about Jane in Broken Promises (page 61). They are shown in a table which indicates where the gaps may come:

I am	*I lack*
1. Concerned, but haven't the facts . . .	G . . . knowledge
2. In possession of the facts but have no authority . . .	A . . . power
3. In a position of power, but it's not really my business . . .	P . . . concern
4. In a position of power, have the knowledge and the concern, but . . .	S . . . drive

A reasonable person might well ask: what can I alone achieve? But what we are trying to point out is that it should be a *team*, not just one reasonable person in isolation who is fighting for the patient.

Still considered against the background of the original incident, such questioning about Tommy's world can lead to constructive thinking, quite apart from the sheer interest of the exercise. Both for the individual whose incident was brought to the group, and as a wider objective for the entire team, it illuminates another aspect of their work, against their own operational problems. It develops also a growing awareness of covert problems, knowledge of which may help the team to avoid the incident in the future.

To some, puzzling over the pathology of their team in an operational situation, it becomes evident that the fourth of these concepts, *drive* is the key factor—and perhaps the most elusive. All the knowledge and concern of the caring professions in a service industry, are of little value unless someone has drive enough to inform, to coordinate, to act. Even power, if clasped possessively to the bosom of the top administrator, is useless to the team (or to the patient)—there must be drive to harness the power. Drive, having apparently little to do with qualifications and skill, let alone with team development, is a concept we appear to know little about; perhaps that is why we waste it with the carelessness of a country experiencing for the first time the vast riches of a newly-discovered mineral.

A group which has travelled this far—or an individual exploring on his own for that matter—will have learned an enormous amount about the pathology of his team, and its vast potential and strength for constructive action planning.

Danger signals

Catch-phrases, like the rattle of machine guns announcing an ambush, pepper the incidents as mechanically as bullets scar a wall. So frequent and pervasive are these sayings, that their value as potential danger signals is evident. Uttered often mechanically, unthinkingly, they accompany every type of incident, signalling problems with roles and relationships, with job satisfaction and priorities, with apathy and frustration. They hang on the lips of juniors and seniors, mothers and matrons, physicians and psychologists, teachers and students.

Recognition that these phrases are sad, unhealthy phrases announcing, like red spots, the presence of disease, could alert a team to take preventive action before disaster occurs. They come from anxious, unhappy, frustrated people . . . and there is a great deal of negative feeling behind them that could well be used creatively to support the team.

Many of the phrases begin with 'I' or (one suspects the royal) 'We'—in itself perhaps signifying that the client has been pushed away from the centre, not deliberately, but by the slag-heap of frustration that has piled up in these individuals.

> 'It's not *my* job!'
> 'I'd rather not ask!'
> 'I'd better not ask . . .'
> 'I'd rather not say.'
> 'I can't very well . . .'
> 'I'm not talking to *her*!'
> 'I'm not looking for trouble!'
> 'Why should I!'

One can feel the apprehension and agony of the student who carefully mixed up the wards' teeth in the night, the discontent of the student nurses crusading with their Cakes for Tea, the uncertainty and fright of the youngster in the Sausage, the insecurity of the armless nurses who crop up everywhere . . .

> 'We haven't time for that . . .'
> 'We haven't time to chat!'
> 'We haven't time for frills!'

Perhaps at first sight and taken at face value, these are reasonable statements. But each, on analysis, suggested to the groups concerned anxiety, unhappiness—energy misspent.

> 'It's not my business.'
> 'Nobody told me.'
> 'What's it got to do with me!'

A feeling of being left out, of bitterness, despondency. 'I wish I were part of a team . . . I wish my opinion mattered!' is what these people are really saying. Could not their indignation be used *for* their clients, instead of against them?

> 'Who does he think he is?'
> 'She should have known . . .'
> 'Let him find out for himself!'

As frequently heard as all the other phrases quoted, the bitterness and resentment, the despondency, the near-vindictiveness are powerfully expressed —and all of them by serious, caring, senior staff.

'Tit-for-tat'
'What's the use!'
'Banging your head against a brick wall . . .'
'*They*!'

Expressive of apathy, hopelessness, frustration, these, too, may be heard at all levels in the hierarchy.

Behind the anxiety and despair, the frustration and discontent, the bitterness and dissatisfaction, one can sense the anger. Apathy, we have said, is a frozen anger, its strength of feeling now unrecognized. It happens, one suspects, where the energy of the young or the new member of a team arrives full of confidence and fresh ideas and crashes into a more than usually rigid administration. Over the years, the energy once used in fighting 'Them', is gradually turned from outward anger to inward apathy. The energy is nonetheless still lying around—an unrecognized strength in a team member.

What seems to us amazing is the power of feeling lying around in these phrases: power which could be used to build and strengthen highly efficient teams but which, neglected, seems to seep into wells of negative energy—trapping the client unwittingly.

The need is twofold: to encourage alertness to these twenty or so danger signals so that the team can avert a serious incident; and to contrive to release the energy behind such phrases, in order to give these individuals the dignity of a creative contribution to the team. We ourselves are constantly recognizing danger signals that we have never heard before: a developing awareness that is a feature of Illuminative Incident Analysis.

Exploration along these lines shows where problems can be recognized, where potential incidents can be spotted, where change can begin. All institutions have their own catchphrases, covering up inadequacies, the bewilderment of a lost child, the fierce hatred of the Old Brigade. All such phrases, as danger signals, indicate not only the need for action, but *where to start the action*. The person who says for instance, 'It's not *my* job', may need support, a shoulder to weep on, a prod in the back or simply a more stimulating project to expand his talents and energies. We would not need to ask such questions as 'Who supports the nurse?' if these signals were heeded and acted upon.

When did you last hear
'it's not *my* job!'
Did *you* feel you were
banging your head . . .?

8. Learning and achievement

Objectives to the Chapter

1. To give illustrations of the early stages of learning—developing awareness

2. To discuss some results of action-learning in the context of Illuminative Incident Analysis.

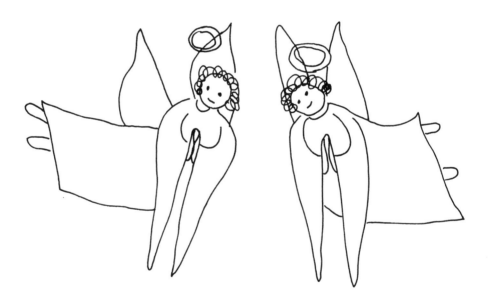

Developing awareness

Action-learning

Any learning process needs time to be absorbed and assimilated. When we are changing, not the material situation, but attitudes, motivation, perception—the deeper aspects of our personality, it is rare to see results overnight. The analysis of Illuminative Incidents is just such a learning process. The temptation, a natural one, is to use it as a material, problem-solving technique: draw your consultant as a tortoise and, bingo, your outpatient queue will dissolve. This was never intended, and, indeed, we have actively discouraged such attempts, believing that, in this process of learning to understand ourselves and our team, absence of immediate results would only lead to frustration and discouragement.

What the technique does is to start a slower, more devious process of changing the perspective of a problem through cartooning it, and so stimulating a new look. As the perspectives alter, so do attitudes begin to change. And the problem, caused in part at any rate, by those faulty attitudes, may no longer seem the same as when it was first revealed by the incident. With fresh perception also comes renewed or redirected motivation.

For instance, in the Four Sons described in chapter 1, the first, obvious problem was the relatives' official complaint about the ward sister, and her consequent bitterness towards them. But she took a fresh look at these relatives when they were drawn as small boys in short pants clasping mother's hand. It was this new look which started to change her attitude towards relatives in general and this, in turn, will change relatives' attitudes towards her, the nurse. Her new, understanding approach in itself will help relatives of future patients to feel less anxious and therefore to be less demanding— and so less likely to precipitate another incident. Her attitude is no longer a negative one of avoiding relatives, but a positive one: 'How best can I support them?'

So, even without any material solutions (such as the handbook for relatives, and regular meetings to discuss their problems with them) the perspective has changed, the ward sister has changed, and her team of nurses will follow her lead. The whole ward will function better, simply because this sister, in the process of analysing her own incident in a vivid way, became aware of the relationship between relatives, patient and herself, and changed in the process. And, having changed herself, she will, ultimately change the bone of contention—relatives.

And so, rather than solving material problems, what we are aiming at is *developing awareness:*

    awareness—of ourselves as individuals
    awareness—of our team
    awareness—of ourselves as others see us
    awareness—of our own hidden potential
    awareness—of the unused assets of the team
    awareness—of the strengths of the grass-roots people.

This is a technique for individual growth and for team development: an opportunity for the only practical and effective way of learning how to work together—learning *from* a current, real situation; and learning *in* a group.

For these reasons we regard this technique as an action-learning process. We are examining a here-and-now problem proposed to the group by one of its members, a problem of personal experience. The group itself decides how to tackle the drawing and where to go next. Looking at the incident and the problem underlying it in this social context within the group, often develops a group feeling that eventually stimulates action. Group learning proliferates ideas; it supports each individual member in his uncertainty; the individual finds more energy, dares to tackle harder goals than he probably could on his own.

Having seen a number of possibilities in the vivid context of a familiar incident, and within the shelter of a group, there comes the inescapable need for the individual to take action. Confronted by himself as seen by other people, the point is reached when only he himself can take the responsibility for doing something about himself.

In this way, the individual is part of a spiral process. First, the group enables him to see and explore the possibilities, in a context in which the negative energy absorbed into the incident has been freed for action. In the process of exploring, he is changed. Next, from his altered position, he can see the situation from a different angle, sees perhaps different problems and other possibilities, and the kind of action required to change the situation. Third, in changing the situation, new features arise and a new awareness develops. Once such awareness is reached, the spiral process flows under its own impetus within the setting of the individual's own team, and action-learning becomes a dynamic and continuous process.

Whether or not the individual is fully conscious of the process, having learned to look at himself—which is the first active step towards developing new attitudes, it is virtually impossible for him not to continue learning and growing. To retreat down the old path becomes difficult, because even if, at a given moment, he has not the courage, or the opportunity to act differently —he is at least now aware of what can and should be done. This awareness, like an uncomfortable itch will pop up again and again in similar situations, when there may be more favourable circumstances or better support from others, and he will be able to act, to learn, to grow and to act again, in the spiral process.

So, developing awareness stimulates action in this way, and further learning will take place—because the individual and members of his team are now likely to be highly sensitive both to people and to situations within the framework of their own operational settings. The process, once started, is one of continuous growth.

Amo, amas, amat

There are two kinds of learning that seem particularly relevant to Illuminative Incident Analysis. The first might be likened to a train reaching its terminus: its destination and the stopping points en route are known and planned. When this kind of learning has been acquired, all that is necessary is to know the rules of how and when to use it. The picture is familiar to us all, of children learning their twice times table, or the Latin scholar ploughing through his verbs and declensions: 'Amo, amas, amat, . . .' This kind of learning plays a valuable part in development, but the knowledge acquired in this way does not necessarily adapt to changing needs.

The second kind of learning is 'kangaroo' learning. As the kangaroo bounds swiftly across the outback, so this type of learner pays little heed to set tracks and predetermined stopping places. It is like the child's game of cumulative leapfrog, when the team leaps over each member in turn. The leader of the moment may take any direction he chooses; the tail of the team is constantly leaping in progression to the front, with the support of every person in front of him until he, in his turn, chooses the direction in which he will lead, and gives his back to his colleagues to lean on and leap over.

The difference between the two types of learning can be likened to that between the vertical and the lateral thinking of Edward de Bono: the one, a style of thinking which always proceeds logically, and the other, a sideways, creative approach which leaps over logic, and which is aware that there is no final stopping place. There is no limit: for each goal achieved sets a fresh goal to be aimed at.

In the practical, everyday context of the team's ability to learn, these two distinct approaches, both of which are necessary, may be described as follows:

> *The look-for-a-rule*, look-for-a-leader, look-for-a-memo, type of approach.
> *The what-needs-to-be-done*? why-not-try-this? what-can-I-myself-do? who-can-join-in? type of approach.

The one is a well-tried, if authoritarian method, where there is always something or someone to take over responsibility (at least, on paper). The other, in sharp contrast, is a questioning, exploratory, perhaps iconoclastic approach where the responsibility is primarily 'I Myself'—for myself *and* others, where teamwork becomes a built-in way of life. It is the difference between:

> 'All you have to do is issue standing orders covering every circumstance' and
> 'Coordination is an attitude of mind.'

The first multi-disciplinary discussion we had, on Peter's Leg (described in chapter 4), nailed it down neatly:

> 'You *want* a set of rules, a magic formula for your client . . . you *need* to develop a sense of responsibility, a feeling of *my* responsibility—for both my client and my colleagues.'

The two approaches are to some extent complementary, and there will always be occasions when members of a team will need to mark time, to refuel and refresh themselves, or perhaps through temporary anxieties to revert to the security of 'amo, amas, amat, . . .'. But growth is like this: it takes place only if we play leapfrog, but it needs a rest on a plateau, to consolidate.

The Thirty-four Per Cent

A small number of people will be able to achieve creative goals immediately. Some will achieve them slowly, with much encouragement from the group: some may get no further than 'amo, amas, amat'. . . We have already referred in chapter 2 to a study in Dallas of student reaction to change and to the Thirty-four Per Cent of a year's intake who were unable to accept an opportunity to explore a new situation, reacting passively, or even violently to an unstructured learning task, and searching frantically for regulations which would force the authorities to teach in the traditional way.

Once encountered, it is easy to recognize a Thirty-four Percenter, and as well to be aware of him for he often has a loud voice. In any large group, this proportion is likely to be found, greeting new ideas negatively and often destructively. Research is currently continuing in the States into the mystery of these unwilling developers: the field is wide open for exploration in this country.

Since growth is such a natural and continuous process, stopping only with death, it puzzles us that such a large number of people are stunted in this way. What is it in our educational system, that can throw up Thirty-four Per Cent of eighteen-year olds who, even at that age, have a need to be taught rather than to learn, and who seem to have lost their natural curiosity? An infant has this natural, restless desire to explore and to learn; a three-year old toddler cannot be stopped from investigating everything within reach. At what age, then, does the transition from the exploratory instinct—without which the human race could not survive, change subtly into the spoon-feeding, 'teach me!' attitude?

If large organizations such as the health and social services (and government departments and industry, for that matter) are to survive they, like the toddler, must explore restlessly. A nation of Thirty-four Percenters would be sterile indeed.

Achievement

We have deliberately kept this section short. Since learning of this kind is an ongoing process, there is no final outcome, and solutions change with changing needs. It is a dynamic activity. And although the teach-me type of learning can be achieved and measured in a matter of hours, there is always a time-lag in assimilating the new ideas implied in an action-learning exercise. Creative social learning is not restricted to time or place: its classroom is the 'shop floor,' or wherever the client is. It cannot always be produced or reproduced on request; it can emerge at any time.

Typology of illuminative incidents

Before illustrating achievements arising out of specific incident analyses, we list below a general outcome of working with this technique over several years. In looking at the most common characteristics, a typology of incidents has emerged—the most frequently found causes of disservice to the patient, or the client:

▶ client not at centre of team's thinking
▶ ignorance and misperception of roles—particularly the 'how does he see me?' concept
▶ lack of teamwork
▶ lack of constructive leadership
▶ apathy.

These are by no means the only characteristics of an incident; they are, so far in our investigations, the major ones. Research is continuing into the minor, but no less frequent, characteristics which may be classified under such sub-headings as:

▶ You can't have *two* things wrong with you!
▶ Tit-for-tat
▶ Ignoring the patient's voice.

But the most striking aspect of all, which we have met somewhere in every single Illuminative Incident, is a disregard for human dignity. Dignity is a right of all human beings; it is the right of all staff at every level—even those below floor level; it is the right of all members of a team, of every relative. Above all, dignity is the unquestionable right of every client and patient.

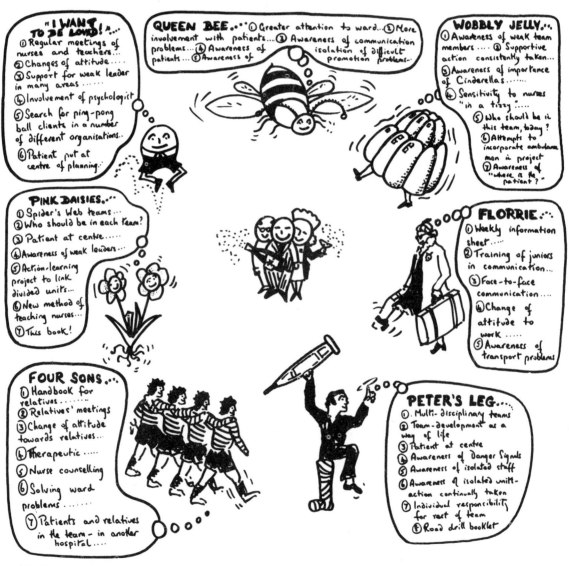

'Action!'

'*Action!*'

We have asked a professional artist (for the first time in this book) to design an illustration of the main achievements in seven particular incidents, chosen either because these groups were followed up over a long period, or because the concepts and cartoons have been widely used for teaching purposes. He has centred the 'Action' illustration (page 104) around the doctor-nurse-patient trio.

It can be seen that the action learning has mainly taken the form of changing attitudes and changes in work habits. In addition, there are some specific products, such as a weekly information sheet and a road-drill booklet.

The most important change is in *sensitivity*. Sensitivity to the Cinderellas, to the Nurse in a Tizzy, to the Wobbly Jelly and to the Leader who Needs to be Loved. These are the perceptions and attitudes which will lead us to seek out many gaps in the service we give our clients, gaps which are not necessarily obvious ones.

Some changes are less tangible, but the effects are nonetheless visible. These are the cathartic and healing processes, where the initial bitterness engendered by the incident has dissolved and the negative energy is now harnessed to constructive attitudes. The Four Sons, perhaps the most dramatic, dissolved the incoherent bitterness of the ward sister and converted it into lasting, constructive concern for relatives and their needs.

It does not matter which incident precipitated this next drawing. It was the last in a series which became more and more primitive, until this childish

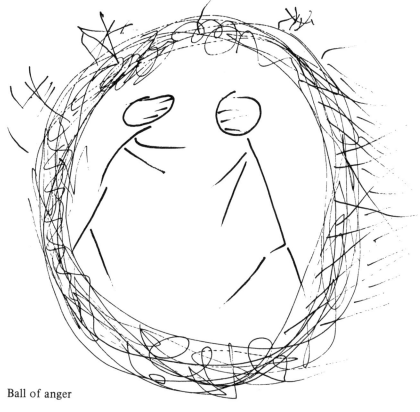

Ball of anger

scribble emerged. The doctor whose incident was being analysed, finally went off into a corner on her own and covered a whole sheet of newsprint with her Ball of Anger. *This* was how she felt about the situation—not what commonsense told her had happened. Like several other scribbled, incoherent illustrations, this was drawn from the stomach. When the doctor finally rejoined the group, she said with a sigh of relief: 'That feels much better!'

It is this therapeutic change, the release of energy for reallocation to constructive action, which we feel is a major outcome of our technique. We said at the beginning that it was not shortage of money, staff or material goods that is the primary problem in the health and social services. It is the unforgivable wastage of human resources which deeply concerns us. We think our technique offers one way of dealing with this.

To underline our point, the Energy Diagram bears repetition here:

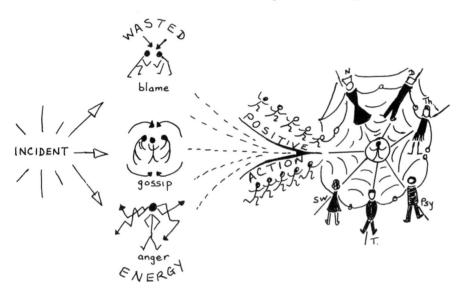

Ideals

In the best of all possible worlds, what sort of benefits would we expect people to find after working on an Illuminative Incident Analysis? We have talked throughout the book of the achievements of various groups and individuals; we have sometimes indicated further possibilities for exploration had time not been limited, or spoken of short demonstration sessions. The Four Sons group spent four main sessions on their incident, at intervals of several weeks, while Ben spent a Sunday morning virtually alone on Cakes for Tea, but brooded about it beforehand and had some tutorial help. What are the greater benefits from a greater time investment and from using several groups of five or six people?

This is a learning situation, and we believe that learning is more meaningful when a group works out its own problems and then gets additional stimulus from reporting back to a larger group. Different groups, like individuals, will naturally progress at different rates of learning—and this is primarily 'kangaroo-type' learning, often with blinding flashes of sudden insight. This, for some people, may be more effective than laborious achievement over several hours, but others may need a gap between sessions.

We have not been able to predict on any occasion how much will be explored, discovered, learned, remembered and acted upon. However, in three or four sessions we would hope that all but the Thirty-four Per Cent would have a better understanding of, and the likelihood of acting upon, much of the following:

Patient or client
More often at the centre of thinking
Considered as part of the team
Concern for 'Tommy-without-me'—(how do I provide for the well-being of my patients when I am no longer there?)

Personal development
Increased awareness of own needs for self-development and personal growth
Greater facility for empathy
Increased sensitivity to needs and roles of others. Consciousness of: How You See Me
Increased energy, channelled positively
Fewer feelings of frustration and impotence
Greater alertness to changing situations and tolerance of change
Ability and drive to search for own questions, to answer such questions as: Who supports the nurse in my team? To consider: Who is the client at this moment of time?—not always clear, for example, in supplies or administrative departments
Insight into and use of danger signals.

Team development
Grasp of what makes a team tick, and insight into own contribution in creating and maintaining such a team
Awareness of the pathology of the team
Awareness and use of organizational danger signals (discussed in the following chapter)
Positive support for weak members of team—and recognition of own patches of weakness
Sensitivity to styles of leadership and to self as a leader
Will look around to see who could contribute to the team.

Communication
Alert to blocks of all types
No longer talking of communication as the central problem.

Illuminative Incidents
Ability to analyse a situation and to spot the gaps in the service to a client
Alert a potentially destructive situation
Creative usage of such situations if they occur.

Actual remedies
As appropriate to a given situation.

We are not suggesting that many of these attributes are not already present, but there should be an increase in awareness and in active use of them. Nor are we suggesting that, magically, four sessions will lead to perfection: it is not easy to change or to accept change. 'Listen to your Cinderellas!' we have advised. But when one of our own Cinderellas comes out with a home truth in front of a group of visitors, it requires a superhuman effort not to revert to hierarchical dignity and an authoritarian stare.

To develop all these facets of insight, awareness and action would be to aspire to Utopia; but they could make a powerful contribution to the formula for a Health Care Plan for any team, for in them is contained all that is necessary for the diagnosis, prevention and cure of the sicknesses that bedevil any organization where groups of people come together for a common purpose.

Amo, amas, amat—
or the kangaroo hop?
A team needs both—
but which are you?
Can *you* play leapfrog?

9. New routes, new hazards

Objective to the chapter

To distinguish both broad issues and the types of block met at the level of involving groups in a new technique which, because it challenges the traditional, 'gloss it over, sweep it under the carpet,' attitudes, may arouse defensive feelings.

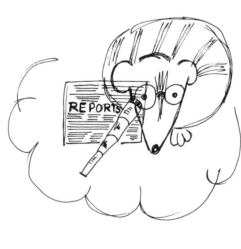

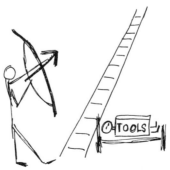

Any kind of exploration, any innovation, is likely to arouse initial opposition, particularly in a hierarchical type of organization. And that resistance is likely to be strong in direct proportion to the need for a fresh look. We have not pretended that this is an easy technique: it is never comfortable for an individual or a group to learn about themselves, for with recognition of their potential and their strength comes responsibility for action. And it is, as one student remarked, often easier to leave things as they are—even when you know they could be better.

To help the innovator, and perhaps to spice the challenge, we have assembled in this chapter some of the problems likely to be met, together with our own experiences. We have then come down to details, and have analysed actual comments made in the course of some hundreds of sessions both in this country and abroad. It is of no use to explore without being aware of the hazards.

Leaving the main highway

Broad pathways

The problems of getting support for this method of team development, which has a certain novelty, are complex and delicate. Sooner or later, a pattern begins to emerge, and phrases heard originally some months before in one setting are echoed and re-echoed by different people, at different levels in the hierarchy, in quite a different place . . . but the words are exactly the same.

Support, of course, implies both initial acceptance of a new method and continued willingness to use it. It implies also support from below, as well as from above; support, too, from one's peers, since no technique can be developed and survive in isolation or without assistance. In getting adequate support, three angles seem particularly prominent:

▶ the problem of authority
▶ the problem of need
▶ the problem of access.

Authority to enter an organization to start a new project, or, indeed, to use a new method within one's own, must be obtained at some point in order to develop and use the experience to the full. It is possible, of course, to do both within one's own department or discipline, or, by using subterfuge, outside it; but this is hardly involving a team in the full, multi-disciplinary sense. The theme of this book is the team, and it is important, therefore, to consider who can sanction the exploration and use of a new technique such as this so that it may be fully used.

Secondly, an unfamiliar way of looking at a team seems more likely to be acceptable if there is a strong need, an urgent problem, a conscious anxiety or specific concern within the organization. In times of fuel crises, the man who invents a petrol-saving gadget will be listened to with some urgency; when fuel is cheap and plentiful, who cares about wastage?

The third angle, the problem of access, is equally important. Access not only to authority, but to that part of the organization which has the facilities and the drive to pursue something new—and to sustain it when things become difficult, as they surely will.

In all three aspects of getting support for this technique, there have been interesting contrasts between the practical problems in one's own organization, and those outside it. And a contrast between the support of the training and education staff, obtained relatively easily, and the difficulty of getting a new method tried and consistently used in day-to-day shop-floor management: in this case, on the ward.

Minor roads

We take first, as a practical example, what happened when we ourselves tried to promote change and introduce Illuminative Incident Analysis in our own hospital. Our route was for us the easiest area of acceptance: the nurse training school.

The problem of authority
Who was it who could give permission for a departure from the accepted syllabus, at that time fairly rigidly structured? Circumstances were fortunate. The nurse training school was in the same building as the psychology department: there were newly-appointed and active heads in both. Both heads were looking for a different approach from straightforward lecturing and discussion; and both respected each other's ideas. The problem melted away at the first meeting.

Access
This was equally simple. Psychology lectures were well-established and covered a two-year period, and at that time there were three entry classes each year. In practice this meant that there were few weeks in the year when a class of students was not available. It was also possible to meet the same class several times and to explore the same incident in great depth. Access, again, was no problem.

Need
The students wanted more realistic lectures which would have, in their opinion, some bearing on what they were doing on the wards. Their feeling was particularly strong on the subject of psychology—which could easily become a technical lecture somewhat remote from the daily life of a student nurse. The technique produced realistic, lively sessions, with material brought by the students *from their world*, developing into topics covering many aspects of the psychology syllabus.

We therefore had all three prerequisites. The two senior people, tutor and psychologist, were fresh to their jobs, conscious of problems and willing to accept the consequences of trying a new approach; and each was sufficiently obstinate to follow her own persuasion without interference from above. Support from below was even more simple. The new method satisfied the students' need for lectures relating to their daily experiences on the ward; it gave them a peep into the attitudes and priorities of those above; it made a welcome break from straight lecturing. Above all, it worked. Fascinating data, entrancing both students and lecturer, began to emerge, and unexpected facets of organization life prompted further exploration. It proved to be a dynamic teaching tool.

The motorway

Any Ulysses has one ability: the inability to remain content with his achievement. The challenge and charm of exploration is this deep discontent. And having seen how lively this technique could be in teaching psychological concepts to young students, it was inevitable to ask: how about management?

Access
This followed a tortuous route which ended again in the field of staff training but this time at both middle and senior management levels.

Starting as an unexpected by-product of a research programme, an account of this team-building technique was first printed as part of the research report and distributed to many disciplines concerned with mental handicap without, so far as can be seen, any response beyond the level of: 'Oh, how fascinating!'

Much later, through a series of personal contacts a demonstration session was arranged (from top level) with an astonished group of nurses who had been expecting a discussion on attitudes, and who found themselves poring over sheets of paper, drawing angels, doctors and devils as they analysed their own Illuminative Incidents. This session ultimately led to these same nurses demonstrating their work to a conference of senior nurse tutors. It was the turning point. Access to middle management courses in teaching hospitals followed soon after, and later, the opportunity to work with senior medical management. As the technique gained recognition, contact with organizations outside the health and social services provided an interesting backcloth to the main setting of this book, indicating the value of the technique in varied settings and at many levels.

Need and authority
The group involved in the demonstration session happened to have a strong need, and they chose two highly emotional incidents to explore. There was continued interest and visible support both from the top, and from an outside organization concerned with another project. The group themselves discovered that it worked—and that it led to constructive action. It had therapeutic benefits, and some of the group continued to use the technique on the ward. Both need and support from authority at all levels existed throughout.

We have found that authority and access to an organization are usually vested in one person in a senior position, having virtual autonomy: in a nurse-training school, someone of, but apart from, the hierarchy; a senior manager in a small unit of a large teaching hospital; outside lecturers, attached to colleges and developing management training; an institute developing management skills in personnel from overseas. In each case they were working with the organizations, but not directly responsible to them—guests, rather than members of the family.

Tutors, college lecturers, organizers of courses—they are people with both authority and access, but people standing slightly apart from the institutions they serve. These staff seem to be vividly aware of needs—particularly of the need to 'take a fresh look at ourselves'. And there also seem to be the people who can openly accept that all may not be well, that critical incidents do occur. They appear less defensive than those from either senior or middle levels who are perhaps more directly concerned with patient, than with staff welfare; and who do not necessarily see the benefit of linking the two together.

Spaghetti junction

Some of the practical difficulties in getting a new method of management education accepted initially have been mentioned as broad factors: authority to try it; access to a suitable group or area of the organization; and the problem of need. This section describes some of the spiky by-roads and misleading road signs we have encountered.

Organizational danger signals

We have taken actual verbatim comments to illustrate the pathology of resistance. They may, by now, be recognized as familiar danger signals: this time, warning us of future perils to the health of the organization, as well as of the individual.

▶ myth of excellence: 'There's no need for such methods here.'
'Such incidents couldn't possibly happen in this organization!'

▶ myth of the busy administrator: 'There's too many meetings already.'
'We haven't time for *that*.'
'It's all talk and no work.'

▶ apathetic involvement: 'Yes, it's very interesting. *You* call a meeting of some sort and discuss it.'
'Yes, you go and try it somewhere . . .'
'Yes, I'll remember it when we have a course/get a room/find a problem/employ a training officer/finish reorganizing/can spare the staff . . .'

▶ inflexible thinking: 'It's not scientific.'
'You don't understand our work.'
'Do *you* know about our procedures?'
'How do you *know* what X thought—you weren't there!'
'You aren't a doctor—you can't know how doctors feel.'
'It's dangerous to imagine how people feel.'

113

▶ negative thinking:	'It shouldn't have happened!' 'Who was responsible—we need to identify *that* person?' 'There's a regulation to cover that!' 'Who was authorized?' 'He should have been there.' 'They should have known.'
▶ vertical thinking:	'Legally, *that* person is responsible.' 'You have to have a medical officer at the top.' 'Better procedures are necessary.' 'More regulations.' 'Double-checks.' 'Counter-signing.' 'More staff.' 'Better job descriptions.' 'More memos.' 'Better communication.'
▶ orthodox thinking:	'Tell me what to do and I'll do it.' 'I'm responsible for my juniors—they cannot be responsible for me.' 'The nurse cannot be responsible for the doctor—or anybody else in the team—they've all got their own jobs to do.'

These then, are the danger signals for the organization as a whole. They are the comfortable alibis of those who resist change. Like our other, personal danger signals, they can also be used to pinpoint problem areas for manager and grass-roots staff alike.

All change!

To the institution, embroiled in the battles and paperwork of change, which is concerned but hypersensitive, throwing aside tradition and yet remaining hierarchical and protective, a technique which might release energy, initiative and drive can be in itself a threat. And it may be that the effort to face something else new and unknown is just too great for those with 'authority' and 'access' to contemplate—however great their need.

It is necessary to have courage and belief in one's convictions in order to withstand the often petty and spiteful, resistance to change, and to winch up the safety curtain hanging between the old and the new. Sadly the paradox of change is that the people who need it most are the least likely to accept it.

Whatever the resistance, the survivor is likely to find that changes have taken place in himself in the process of innovation, and that he has learned a little more of who and what he is. No mean achievement.

You, an individual interested in developing managers, in understanding teamwork, in initiating change, now know the hazards of the journey. But it is, nonetheless, an exciting, challenging, rewarding exercise. There is always someone who acts as a catalyst to the group, infecting the rest with enthusiasm: and always some delightful drawings like those we have shown in this book. They were all done by ordinary people, learning to work in a team.

If you ever doubt the need for you to get involved, just contemplate this comment from a student nurse in her third year, made at the end of a series of ordinary discussions on roles, attitudes and job satisfaction:

'Yes dear, it's all been very interesting,
and
we all agree with everything you say—
but
what's it got to do with us!'

Could it be that *all* professional training, whether nursing or medical, social work or administrative, technical or engineering, should begin by deliberately teaching the skills of team-building, leaving the technical skills of each profession until each has learned his duty towards, and his dependence upon, the other members of his team? Should we not all learn about ourselves, before working on . . . with . . . for . . . others?

Will you remember
Illuminative Incident Analysis
when . . .?
or
Will you act
now?

10. Conclusions

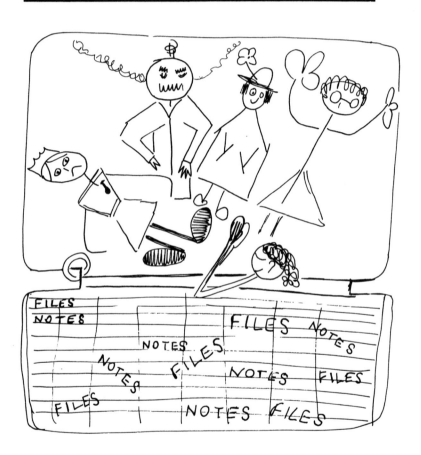

Verbatim discussion

Senior nurse: 'No one seems to have bothered to tell the patient what was happening. Patients are passed over as if they had no interest in things.'

Administrator: 'How do *we* know what the patient felt?'

Social worker:	'Patients *are* frightened—you only have to look at them. They should be part of the team.'
Consultant:	'Patient involvement? Yes, of course. But the hospital staff are too busy, there is no time.'
Ward sister:	'Some doctors find the time.'
Administrator:	'Perhaps the junior doctors have not been instructed on how to talk to the patients?'
Tutor:	'Perhaps the doctor was shy.'
Engineer:	'He can't have been shy—he's a consultant.'

This conversation occurred while discussing the drawings and cartoons that these staff had done in their various groups as a means of exploring some Illuminative Incidents personally experienced by a member of each one. Both top and middle management were represented. The dialogue is reported verbatim, from the full session.

The exchange of opinions shows a nice mixture of vertical and lateral thinking, of sensitive awareness of problems and attitudes, of concern for patients' needs—and almost unbelievable blindness to the issues. 'Patient involvement? Yes, of course. But . . .'

It sums up our thesis.

Who is our client? Where is our client? What does he feel? How can we help? How can we help and support our colleagues? What do they feel and how do they see us?

It is in order to present these issues in startling clarity and to stimulate fresh thinking of a kind that will involve a sequence of action and learning, and further action, that we use Illuminative Incident Analysis. It is a simple technique, at one level: everyone knows of a client who got a raw deal of some kind; everyone can draw pin men; everyone knows his own corner of his own organization and is eager to display his knowledge. Drawing the situation gets a group working together in a relaxed fashion, it's a fresh way of looking at things, it's fun. Exploring the broader issues that lie behind lack of communication, of coordination, of teamwork can be taken to any depth the group and tutor wish.

Our technique draws out such attitudes partly because we use, as a starting point, a highly emotional occurrence, an incident personal to one member of the study group. Most people care about their clients, and care deeply. But we cut discussion to a minimum. Expressing feelings about the incident in drawings and cartoons is a safe and even humorous exercise which, despite its apparent simplicity, reveals attitudes, motives, role perception and the state of team-development, in a highly creative learning situation. It is an opportunity to explore in a social group, and an opportunity for dispelling anger, bitterness and fear.

Incidents, like the visible tip of the iceberg, conceal the hidden depths that are dangerous to the welfare of a healthy team—for teams, like individuals, can fall sick. Depths such as:

▶ mistaken, misguided, misinterpreted attitudes
▶ ill-perceived roles

- ▶ the frustration, the anger, the apathy
- ▶ the misdirected energy
- ▶ the under-used human potential

All organizations, of whatever kind, have incidents lying around like scarlet-skinned sunbathers on a Mediterranean beach. All organizations, of whatever kind, waste human resources. None can afford to.

This technique is applicable in any place where groups come together; we have restricted the examples in this book to the health and social services because this is where we happen to work.

With reorganizations, redistribution and the current speed of change, it is going to be even more vital in the future to have integrated teams working well together at all levels, capable of dealing with expanding and changing roles. It is the right of all of us, as members of a team, to develop and grow in our jobs and to use to the full our energy and skills; to give as well as to take. This is one way of discovering how.

Why wait for the disaster of the Four Sons—
or the frustration of Cakes for Tea?
Why wait for an inquiry, a scandal,
or a young student giving up her career
in an understaffed profession,
before taking action?

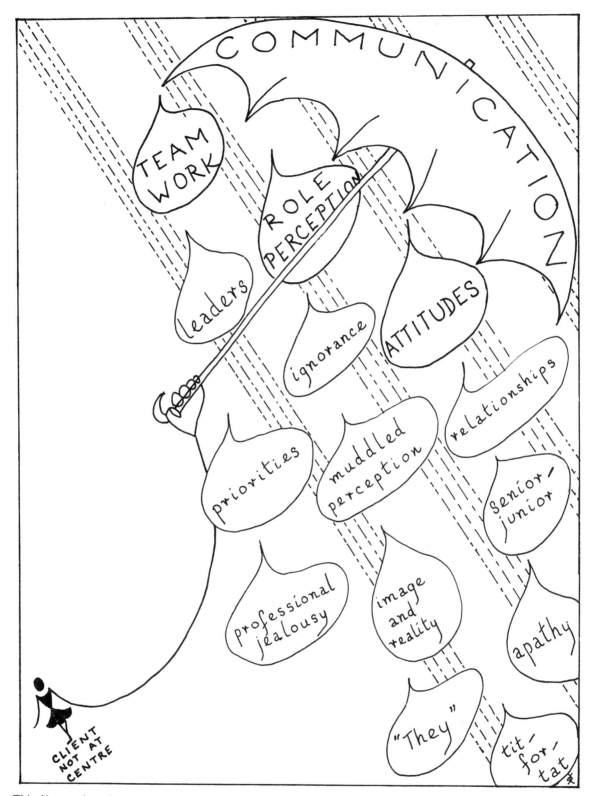

This diagram broadly summarizes our attempts throughout this book to explore the deeper problems of communication in an organization. It shows some of the concepts we have found lurking beneath the protective umbrella term 'communication'.

Index

(Numbers in bold type refer to the major reference)

Printed by William Clowes & Sons Ltd., London, Colchester and Beccles.